Meals for Your Mediterranean Diet

Improve Your Daily Meals with These Super-Tasty Recipes

America Best Recipes

Table of contents

Salmon and Mango Mix

Preparation Time: 10 minutes

Cooking Time: 25 minutes

Servings: 2

Ingredients:

- 2 salmon fillets, skinless and boneless
- Salt and pepper to the taste
- 2 tbsp. olive oil
- 2 garlic cloves, minced
- 2 mangos, peeled and cubed
- 1 red chili, chopped
- 1 small piece ginger, grated
- Juice of 1 lime
- 1 tbsp. cilantro, chopped

Directions:

1. In a roasting pan, combine the salmon with the oil, garlic and the rest of the ingredients except the cilantro, toss, introduce in the oven at 350°F and bake for 25 minutes.
2. Divide everything between plates and serve with the cilantro sprinkled on top.

Nutrition: Calories 251, Fat 15.9g, Fiber 5.9g, Carbs 26.4g, Protein 12.4g

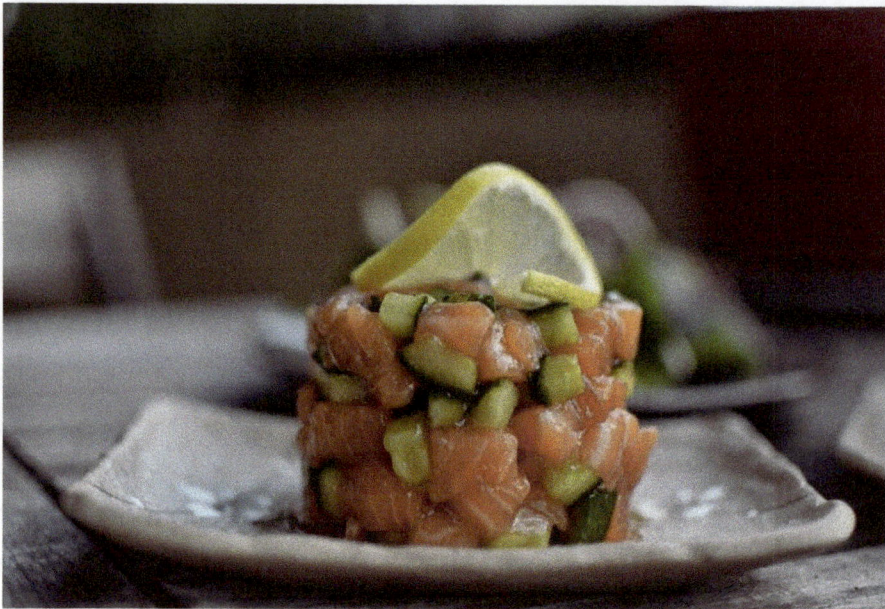

Salmon and Creamy Endives

Preparation Time: 10 minutes

Cooking Time: 15 minutes

Servings: 4

Ingredients:

- 4 salmon fillets, boneless
- 2 endives, shredded
- Juice of 1 lime
- Salt and black pepper to the taste
- ¼ cup chicken stock
- 1 cup Greek yogurt
- ¼ cup green olives pitted and chopped
- ¼ cup fresh chives, chopped
- 3 tbsp. olive oil

Directions:

1. Heat up a pan with half of the oil over medium heat, add the endives and the rest of the ingredients except the chives and the salmon, toss, cook for 6 minutes and divide between plates.
2. Heat up another pan with the rest of the oil, add the salmon, season with salt and pepper, cook for

4 minutes on each side, add next to the creamy endives mix, sprinkle the chives on top and serve.

Nutrition: Calories 266, Fat 13.9g, Fiber 11.1g, Carbs 23.8g, Protein 17.5g

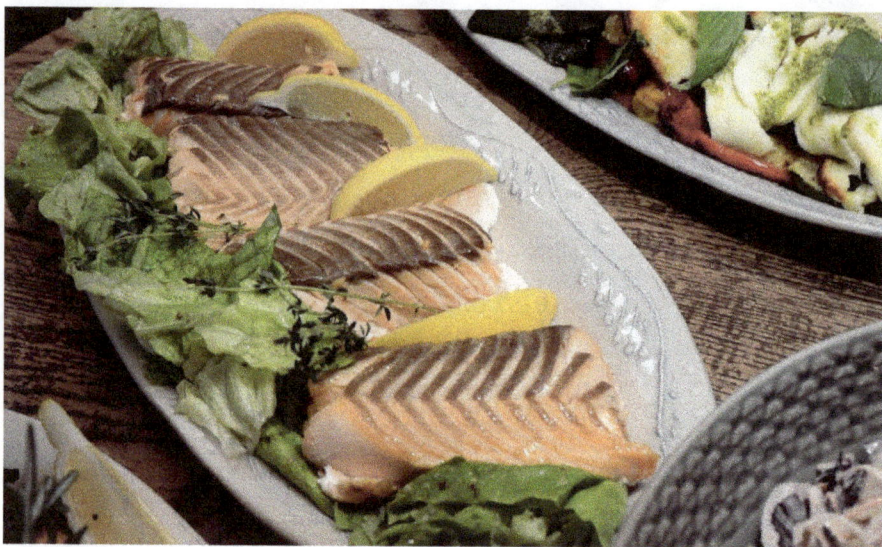

Trout and Tzatziki Sauce

Preparation Time: 10 minutes

Cooking Time: 10 minutes

Servings: 4

Ingredients:

- Juice of ½ lime
- Salt and black pepper to the taste
- 1 and ½ tsp. coriander, ground
- 1 tsp. garlic, minced
- 4 trout fillets, boneless
- 1 tsp. sweet paprika
- 2 tbsp. avocado oil
- For the sauce:
- 1 cucumber, chopped
- 4 garlic cloves, minced
- 1 tbsp. olive oil
- 1 tsp. white vinegar
- 1 and ½ cups Greek yogurt
- A pinch of salt and white pepper

Directions:

1. Heat up a pan with the avocado oil over medium-high heat, add the fish, salt, pepper, lime juice, 1 tsp. garlic and the paprika, rub the fish gently and cook for 4 minutes on each side.
2. In a bowl, combine the cucumber with 4 garlic cloves and the rest of the ingredients for the sauce and whisk well.
3. Divide the fish between plates, drizzle the sauce all over and serve with a side salad.

Nutrition: Calories 393,

Fat 18.5g,

Fiber 6.5g,

Carbs 18.3g,

Protein 39.6g

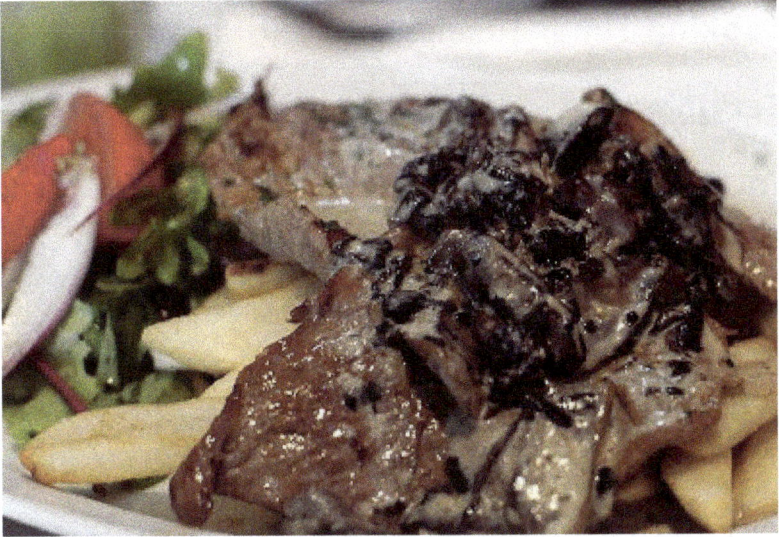

Parsley Trout and Capers

Preparation Time: 10 minutes

Cooking Time: 10 minutes

Servings: 4

Ingredients:

- 4 trout fillets, boneless
- 3 oz. tomato sauce
- A handful parsley, chopped
- 2 tbsp. olive oil
- Salt and black pepper to the taste

Directions:

1. Heat up a pan with the oil over medium-high heat, add the fish, salt and pepper and cook for 3 minutes on each side.
2. Add the rest of the ingredients, cook everything for 4 minutes more.
3. Divide everything between plates and serve.

Nutrition: Calories 308, Fat 17g, Fiber 1g, Carbs 3g, Protein 16g

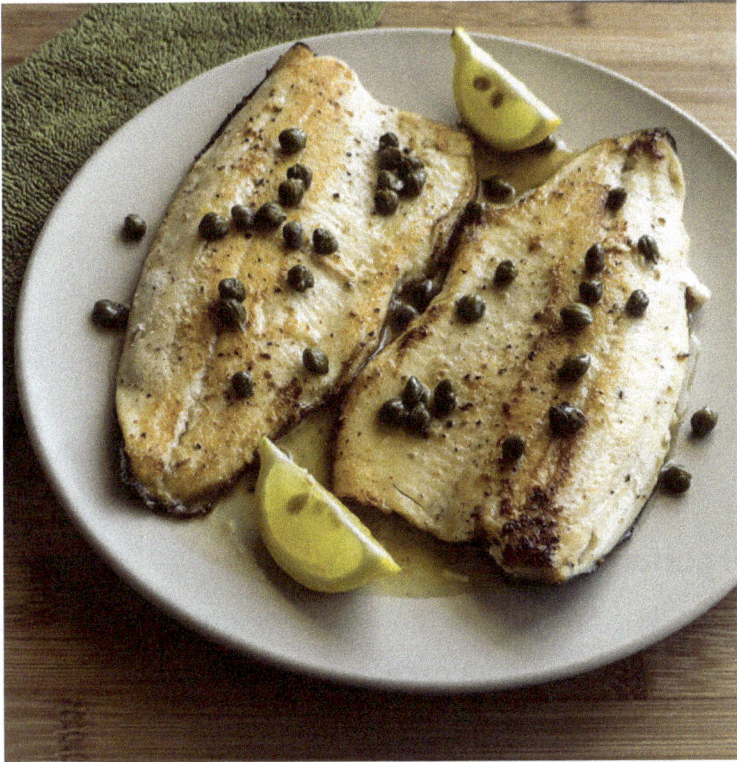

Baked Trout and Fennel

Preparation Time: 10 minutes

Cooking Time: 22 minutes

Servings: 4

Ingredients:

- 1 fennel bulb, sliced
- 2 tbsp. olive oil
- 1 yellow onion, sliced
- 3 tsp. Italian seasoning
- 4 rainbow trout fillets, boneless
- ¼ cup panko breadcrumbs
- ½ cup kalamata olives, pitted and halved
- Juice of 1 lemon

Directions:

1. Spread the fennel the onion and the rest of the ingredients except the trout and the breadcrumbs on a baking sheet lined with parchment paper, toss them and cook at 400°F for 10 minutes.
2. Add the fish dredged in breadcrumbs and seasoned with salt and pepper and cook it at 400°F for 6 minutes on each side.
3. Divide the mix between plates and serve.

Nutrition: Calories 306, Fat 8.9g, Fiber 11.1g, Carbs 23.8g, Protein 14.5g

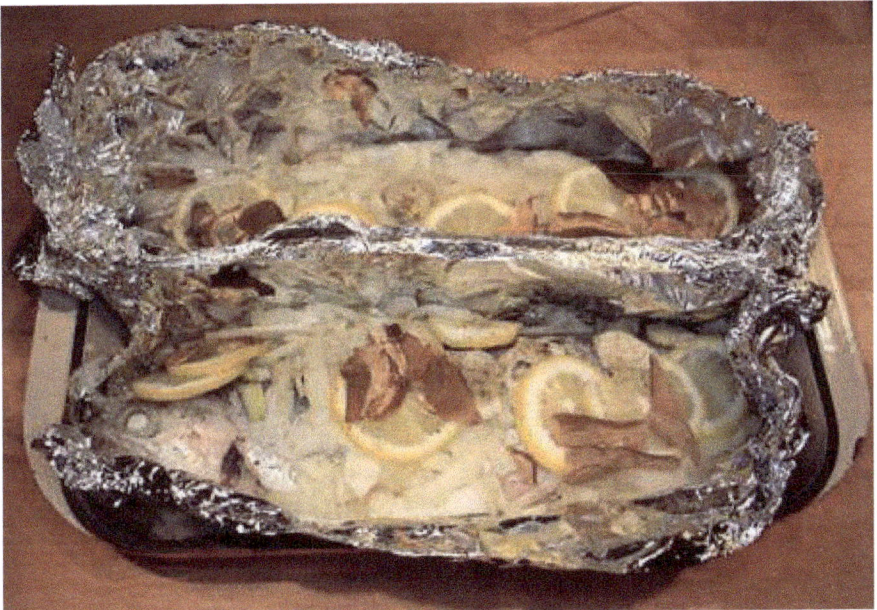

Lemon Rainbow Trout

Preparation Time: 10 minutes

Cooking Time: 15 minutes

Servings: 2

Ingredients:

- 2 rainbow trout
- Juice of 1 lemon
- 3 tbsp. olive oil
- 4 garlic cloves, minced
- A pinch of salt and black pepper

Directions:

1. Line a baking sheet with parchment paper, add the fish and the rest of the ingredients and rub.
2. Bake at 400°F for 15 minutes, divide between plates and serve with a side salad.

Nutrition: Calories 321, Fat 19g, Fiber 5g, Carbs 6g, Protein 35g

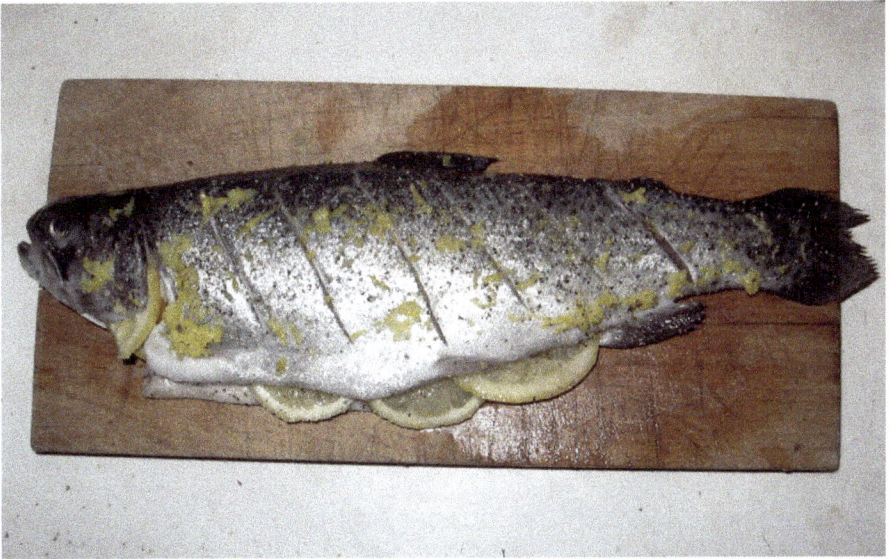

Trout and Peppers Mix

Preparation Time: 10 minutes

Cooking Time: 20 minutes

Servings: 4

Ingredients:

- 4 trout fillets, boneless
- 2 tbsp. kalamata olives, pitted and chopped
- 1 tbsp. capers, drained
- 2 tbsp. olive oil
- A pinch of salt and black pepper
- 1 and ½ tsp. chili powder
- 1 yellow bell pepper, chopped
- 1 red bell pepper, chopped
- 1 green bell pepper, chopped

Directions:

1. Heat up a pan with the oil over medium-high heat, add the trout, salt and pepper and cook for 10 minutes.
2. Flip the fish, add the peppers and the rest of the ingredients, cook for 10 minutes more, divide the whole mix between plates and serve.

Nutrition: Calories 572, Fat 17.4g, Fiber 6g, Carbs 71g, Protein 33.7g

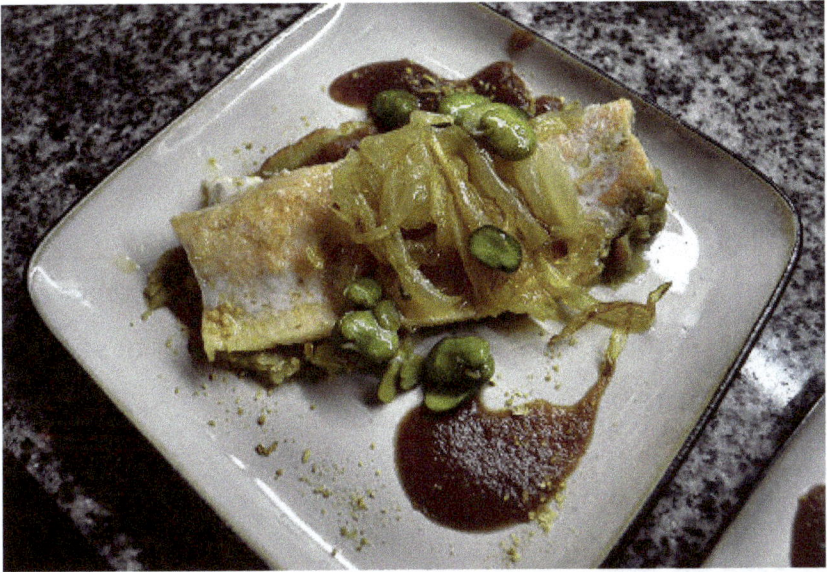

Banana Shake Bowls

Preparation Time: 5 minutes

Cooking Time: 0 minutes

Servings: 4

Ingredients:

- 4 medium bananas, peeled
- 1 avocado, peeled, pitted and mashed
- ¾ cup almond milk
- ½ tsp. vanilla extract

Directions:

1. In a blender, combine the bananas with the avocado and the other ingredients, pulse, divide into bowls and keep in the fridge until serving.

Nutrition:

Calories 185

Fat 4.3g

Carbs 6g

Protein 6.45g

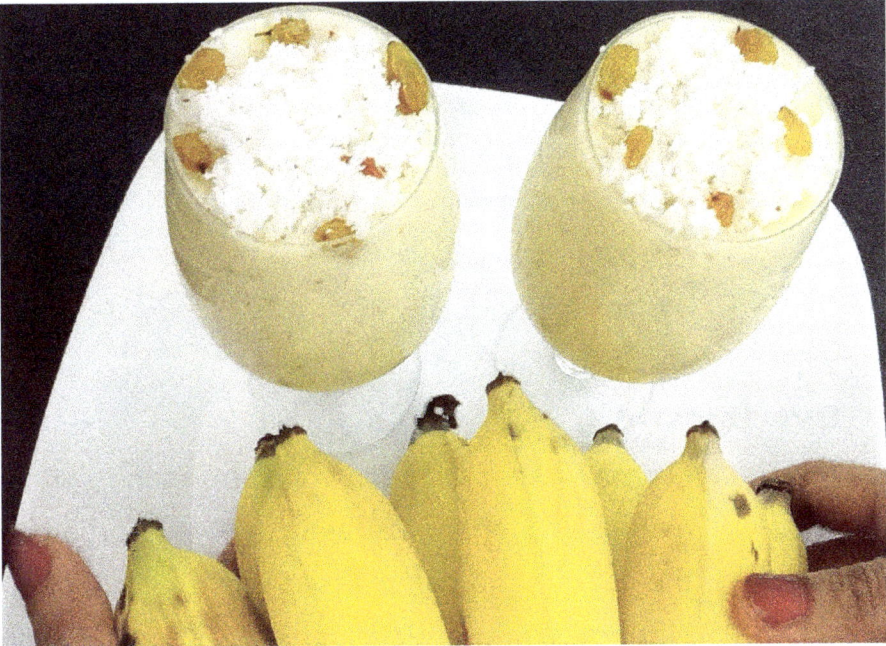

Cold Lemon Squares

Preparation Time: 30 minutes

Cooking Time: 0 minutes

Servings: 4

Ingredients:

- 1 cup avocado oil+ a drizzle
- 2 bananas, peeled and chopped
- 1 tbsp. honey
- ¼ cup lemon juice
- A pinch of lemon zest, grated

Directions:

1. In your food processor, mix the bananas with the rest of the ingredients, pulse well and spread on the bottom of a pan greased with a drizzle of oil.
2. Introduce in the fridge for 30 minutes, slice into squares and serve.

Nutrition:

Calories 136g

Fat 11.2g

Carbs 7g

Protein 1.1g

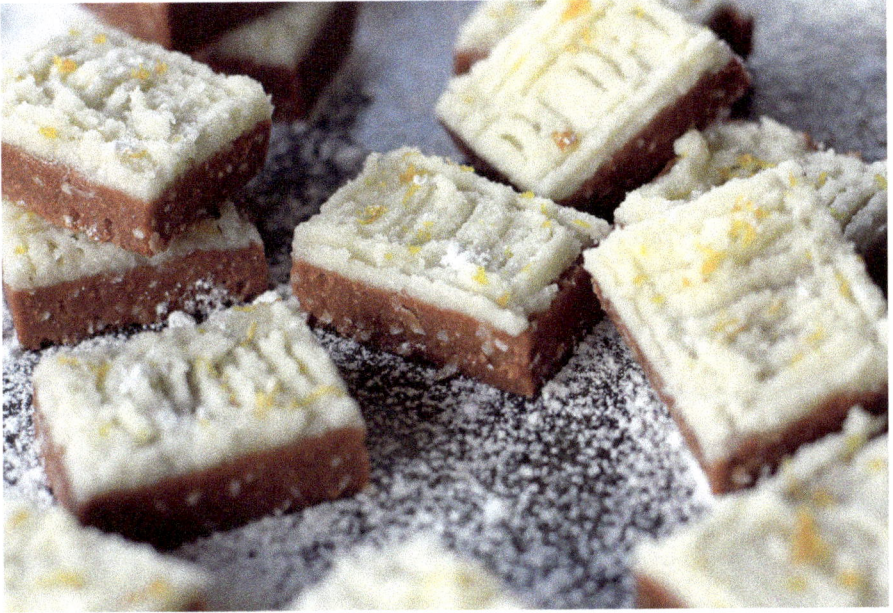

Blackberry and Apples Cobbler

Preparation Time: 10 minutes

Cooking Time: 30 minutes

Servings: 6

Ingredients:

- ¾ cup stevia
- 6 cups blackberries
- ¼ cup apples, cored and cubed
- ¼ tsp. baking powder
- 1 tbsp. lime juice
- ½ cup almond flour
- ½ cup water
- 3 and ½ tbsp. avocado oil
- Cooking spray

Directions:

1. In a bowl, mix the berries with half of the stevia and lemon juice, sprinkle some flour all over, whisk and pour into a baking dish greased with cooking spray.
2. In another bowl, mix flour with the rest of the sugar, baking powder, the water and the oil, and stir the whole thing with your hands.
3. Spread over the berries, introduce in the oven at 375°Fand bake for 30 minutes.

4. Serve warm.

Nutrition:

 Calories 221

Fat 6.3g

Carbs 6g

Protein 9g

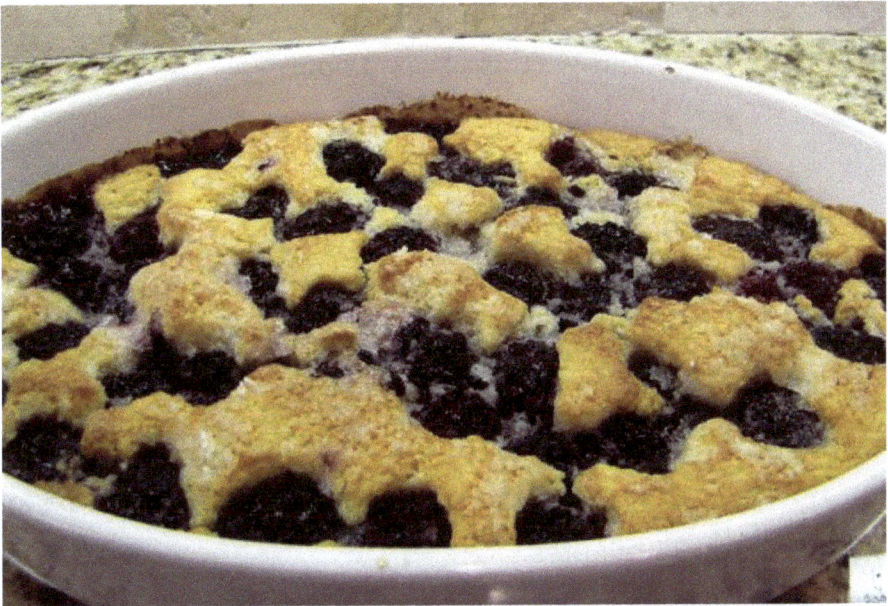

Black Tea Cake

Preparation Time: 10 minutes

Cooking Time: 35 minutes

Servings: 8

Ingredients:

- 6 tbsp. black tea powder
- 2 cups almond milk, warmed up
- 1 cup avocado oil
- 2 cups stevia
- 4 eggs
- 2 tsp. vanilla extract
- 3 and ½ cups almond flour
- 1 tsp. baking soda
- 3 tsp. baking powder

Directions:

1. In a bowl, combine the almond milk with the oil, stevia and the rest of the ingredients and whisk well.
2. Pour this into a cake pan lined with parchment paper, introduce in the oven at 350°F and bake for 35 minutes.
3. Leave the cake to cool down, slice and serve.

Nutrition:

Calories 200

Fat 6.4g

Carbs 6.5g

Protein 5.4g

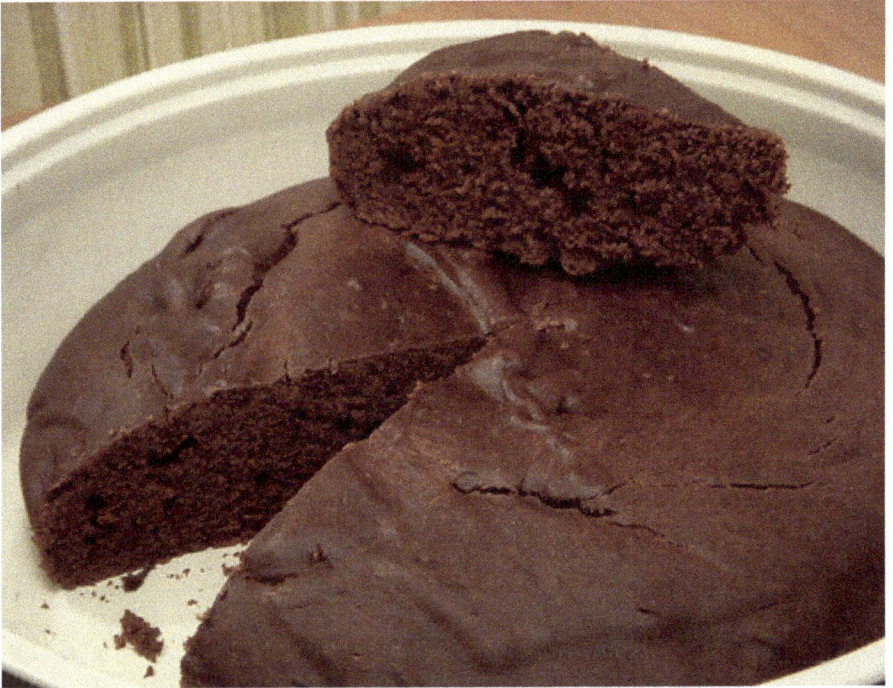

Green Tea and Vanilla Cream

Preparation Time: 2 hours

Cooking Time: 0 minutes

Servings: 4

Ingredients:

- 14 oz. almond milk, hot
- 2 tbsp. green tea powder
- 14 oz. heavy cream
- 3 tbsp. stevia
- 1 tsp. vanilla extract
- 1 tsp. gelatin powder

Directions:

1. In a bowl, combine the almond milk with the green tea powder and the rest of the ingredients, whisk well, cool down, divide into cups and keep in the fridge for 2 hours before serving.

Nutrition:

Calories 120

Fat 3g

Carbs 7g

Protein 4g

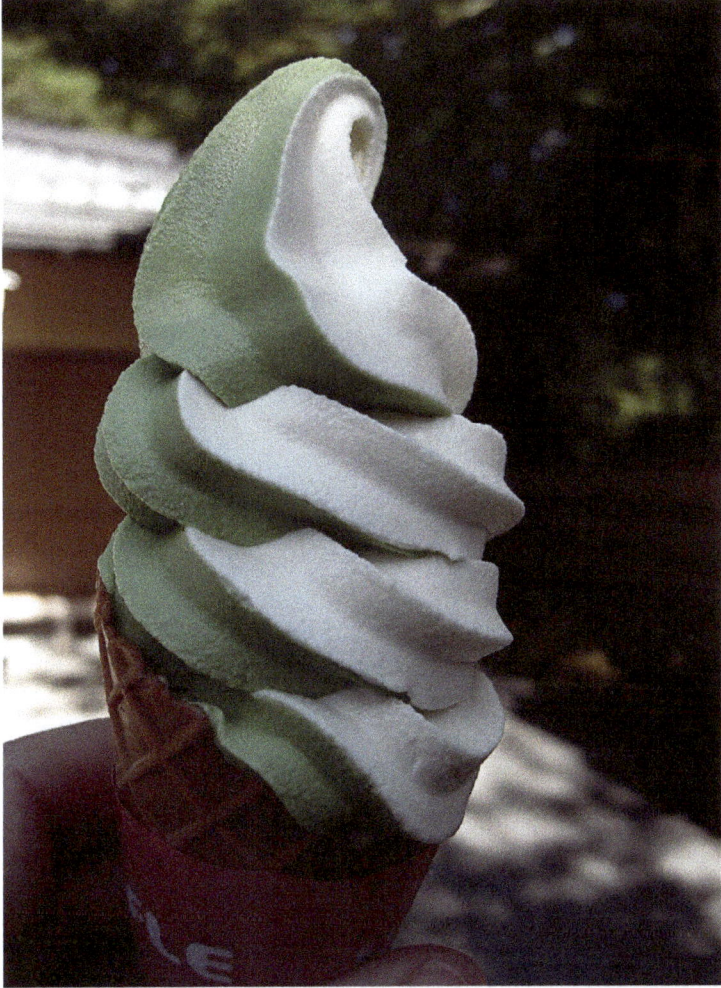

Figs Pie

Preparation Time: 10 minutes

Cooking Time: 1 hour

Servings: 8

Ingredients:

- ½ cup stevia
- 6 figs, cut into quarters
- ½ tsp. vanilla extract
- 1 cup almond flour
- 4 eggs, whisked

Directions:

1. Spread the figs on the bottom of a springform pan lined with parchment paper.
2. In a bowl, combine the other ingredients, whisk and pour over the figs,
3. Bake at 375 digress F for 1 hour, flip the pie upside down when it's done and serve.

Nutrition:

Calories 200

Fat 4.4g

Carbs 7.6g

Protein 8g

Cherry Cream

Preparation Time: 2 hours

Cooking Time: 0 minutes

Servings: 4

Ingredients:

- 2 cups cherries, pitted and chopped
- 1 cup almond milk
- ½ cup whipping cream
- 3 eggs, whisked
- 1/3 cup stevia
- 1 tsp. lemon juice
- ½ tsp. vanilla extract

Directions:

1. In your food processor, combine the cherries with the milk and the rest of the ingredients, pulse well, divide into cups and keep in the fridge for 2 hours before serving.

Nutrition:

Calories 200

Fat 4.5g

Carbs 5.6g

Protein 3.4g

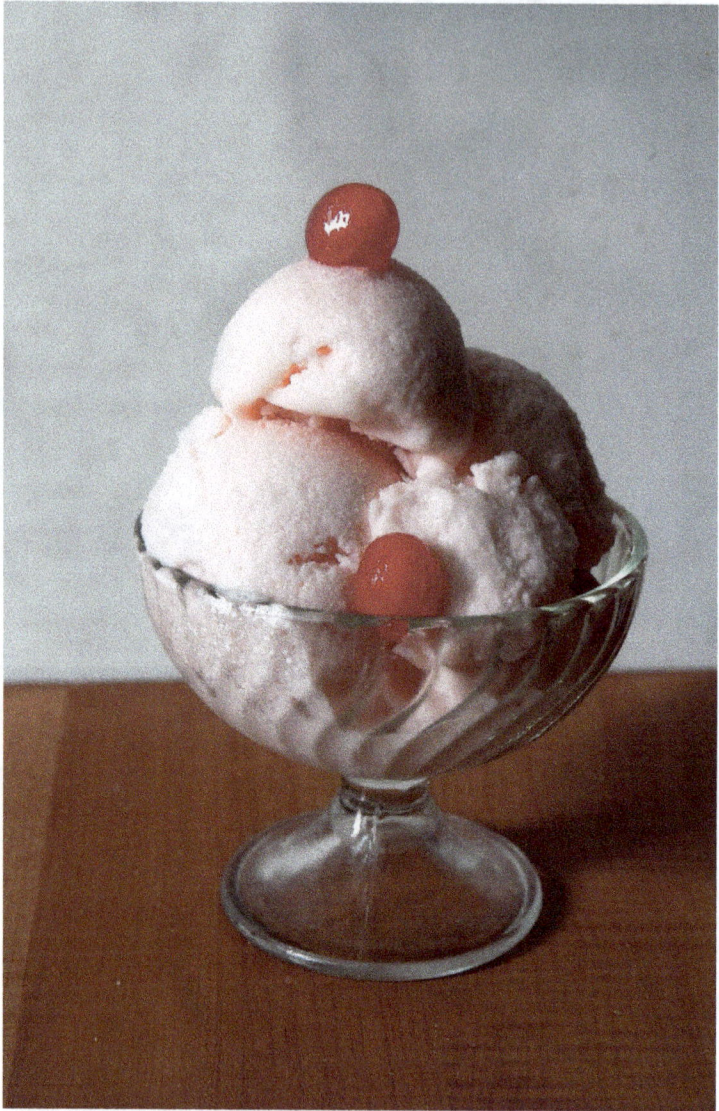

Strawberries Cream

Preparation Time: 10 minutes

Cooking Time: 20 minutes

Servings: 4

Ingredients:

- ½ cup stevia
- 2 lb. strawberries, chopped
- 1 cup almond milk
- Zest of 1 lemon, grated
- ½ cup heavy cream
- 3 egg yolks, whisked

Directions:

1. Heat up a pan with the milk over medium-high heat, add the stevia and the rest of the ingredients, whisk well, simmer for 20 minutes, divide into cups and serve cold.

Nutrition:

Calories 152

Fat 4.4g

Carbs 5.1g

Protein 0.8g

Apples and Plum Cake

Preparation Time: 10 minutes

Cooking Time: 40 minutes

Servings: 4

Ingredients:

- 7 oz. almond flour
- 1 egg, whisked
- 5 tbsp. stevia
- 3 oz. warm almond milk
- 2 lb. plums, pitted and cut into quarters
- 2 apples, cored and chopped
- Zest of 1 lemon, grated
- 1 tsp. baking powder

Directions:

1. In a bowl, mix the almond milk with the egg, stevia, and the rest of the ingredients except the cooking spray and whisk well.
2. Grease a cake pan with the oil, pour the cake mix inside, introduce in the oven and bake at 350°F for 40 minutes.
3. Cool down, slice and serve.

Nutrition:

Calories 209

Fat 6.4g

Carbs 8g

Protein 6.6g

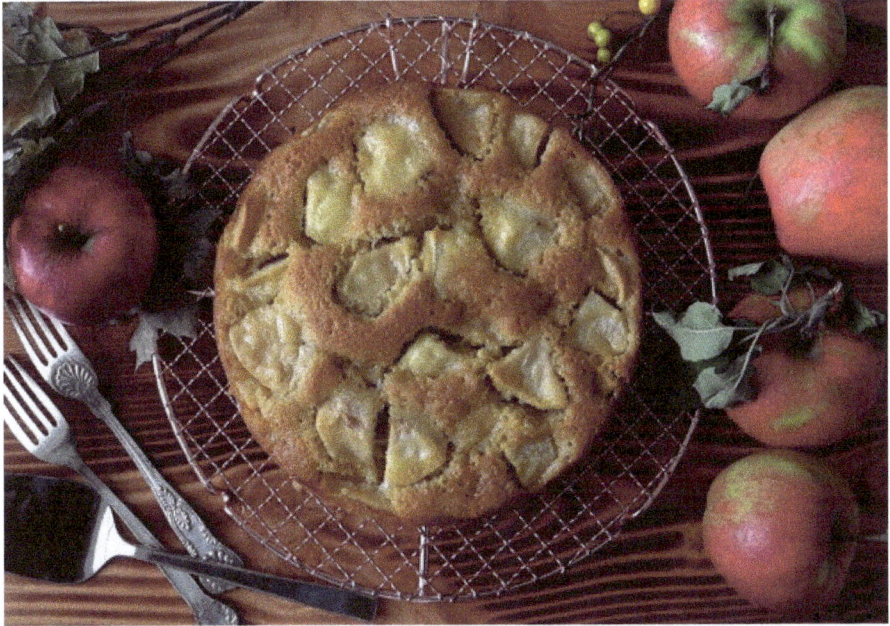

Cinnamon Chickpeas Cookies

Preparation Time: 10 minutes

Cooking Time: 20 minutes

Servings: 12

Ingredients:

- 1 cup canned chickpeas, drained, rinsed and mashed
- 2 cups almond flour
- 1 tsp. cinnamon powder
- 1 tsp. baking powder
- 1 cup avocado oil
- ½ cup stevia
- 1 egg, whisked
- 2 tsp. almond extract
- 1 cup raisins
- 1 cup coconut, unsweetened and shredded

Directions:

1. In a bowl, combine the chickpeas with the flour, cinnamon and the other ingredients, and whisk well until you obtain a dough.
2. Scoop tbsp. of dough on a baking sheet lined with parchment paper, introduce them in the oven at 350°F and bake for 20 minutes.
3. Leave them to cool down for a few minutes and serve.

Nutrition:

Calories 200

Fat 4.5g

Carbs 9.5g

Protein 2.4g

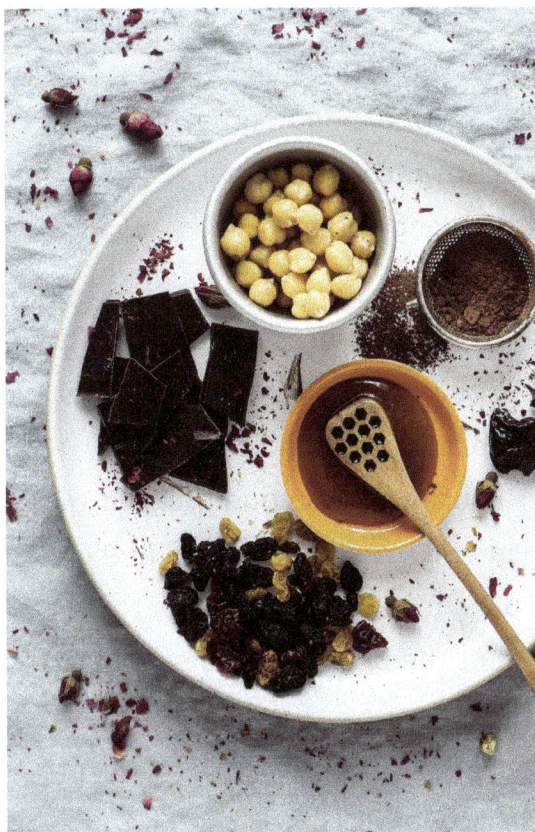

Cocoa Brownies

Preparation Time: 10 minutes

Cooking Time: 20 minutes

Servings: 8

Ingredients:

- 30 oz. canned lentils, rinsed and drained
- 1 tbsp. honey
- 1 banana, peeled and chopped
- ½ tsp. baking soda
- 4 tbsp. almond butter
- 2 tbsp. cocoa powder
- Cooking spray

Directions:

1. In a food processor, combine the lentils with the honey and the other ingredients except the cooking spray and pulse well.
2. Pour this into a pan greased with cooking spray, spread evenly, introduce in the oven at 375°F and bake for 20 minutes.
3. Cut the brownies and serve cold.

Nutrition:

Calories 200

Fat 4.5g

Carbs 8.7g

Protein 4.3g

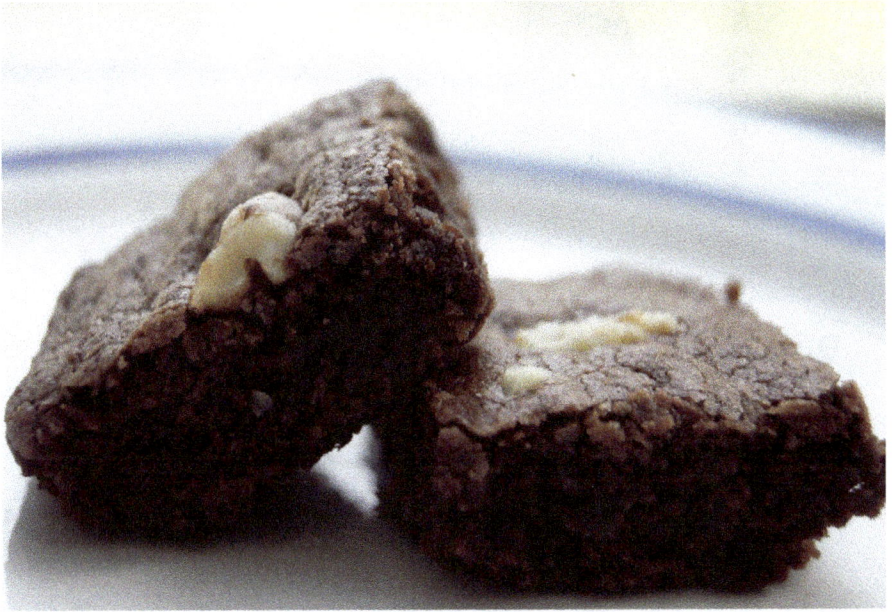

Cardamom Almond Cream

Preparation Time: 30 minutes

Cooking Time: 0 minutes

Servings: 4

Ingredients:

- Juice of 1 lime
- ½ cup stevia
- 1 and ½ cups water
- 3 cups almond milk
- ½ cup honey
- 2 tsp. cardamom, ground
- 1 tsp. rose water
- 1 tsp. vanilla extract

Directions:

1. In a blender, combine the almond milk with the cardamom and the rest of the ingredients, pulse well, divide into cups and keep in the fridge for 30 minutes before serving.

Nutrition:

Calories 283

Fat 11.8g

Carbs 4.7g

Protein 7.1g

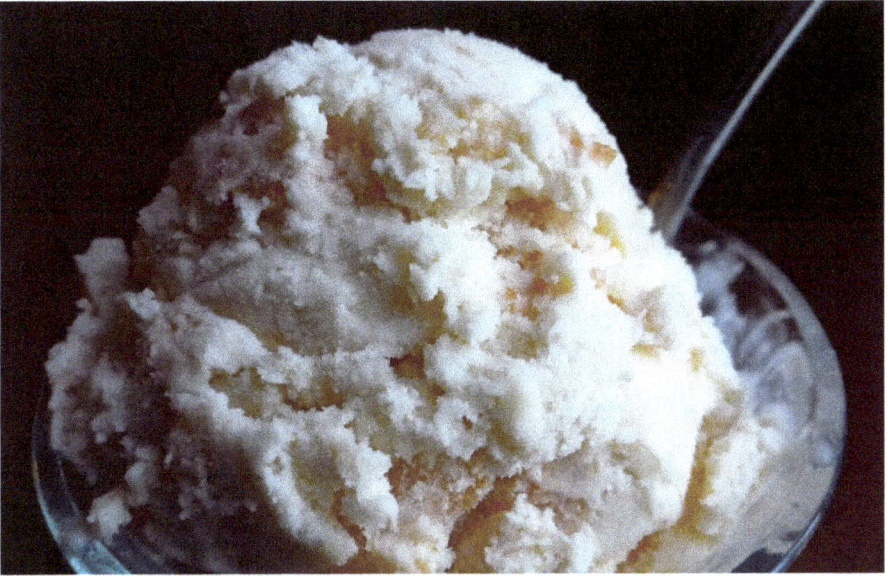

Banana Cinnamon Cupcakes

Preparation Time: 10 minutes

Cooking Time: 20 minutes

Servings: 4

Ingredients:

- 4 tbsp. avocado oil
- 4 eggs
- ½ cup orange juice
- 2 tsp. cinnamon powder
- 1 tsp. vanilla extract
- 2 bananas, peeled and chopped
- ¾ cup almond flour
- ½ tsp. baking powder
- Cooking spray

Directions:

2. In a bowl, combine the oil with the eggs, orange juice and the other ingredients except the cooking spray, whisk well, pour in a cupcake pan greased with the cooking spray, introduce in the oven at 350°F and bake for 20 minutes.

3. Cool the cupcakes down and serve.

Nutrition:

Calories 142

Fat 5.8g

Carbs 5.7g

Protein 1.6g

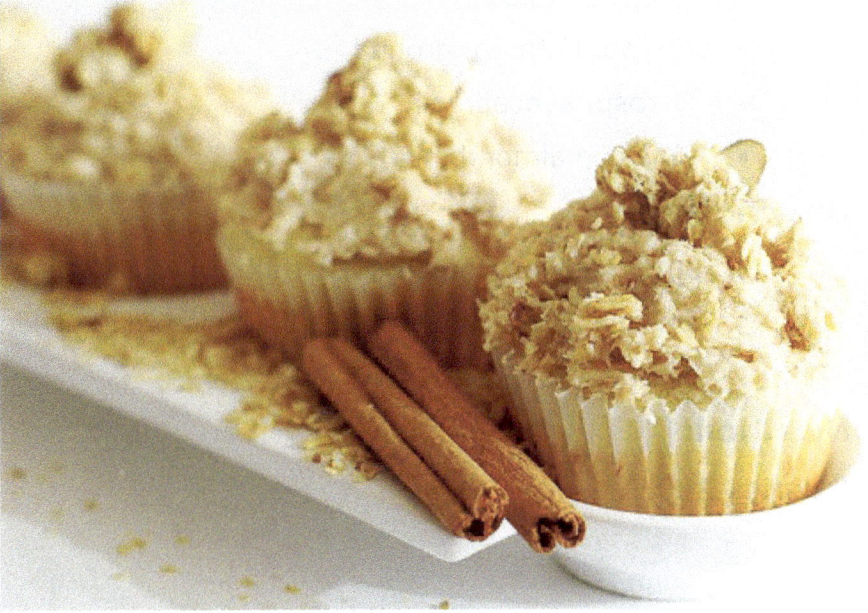

Rhubarb and Apples Cream

Preparation Time: 10 minutes

Cooking Time: 0 minutes

Servings: 6

Ingredients:

- 3 cups rhubarb, chopped
- 1 and ½ cups stevia
- 2 eggs, whisked
- ½ tsp. nutmeg, ground
- 1 tbsp. avocado oil
- 1/3 cup almond milk

Directions:

1. In a blender, combine the rhubarb with the stevia and the rest of the ingredients, pulse well, divide into cups and serve cold.

Nutrition:

Calories 200

Fat 5.2g

Carbs 7.6g

Protein 2.5g

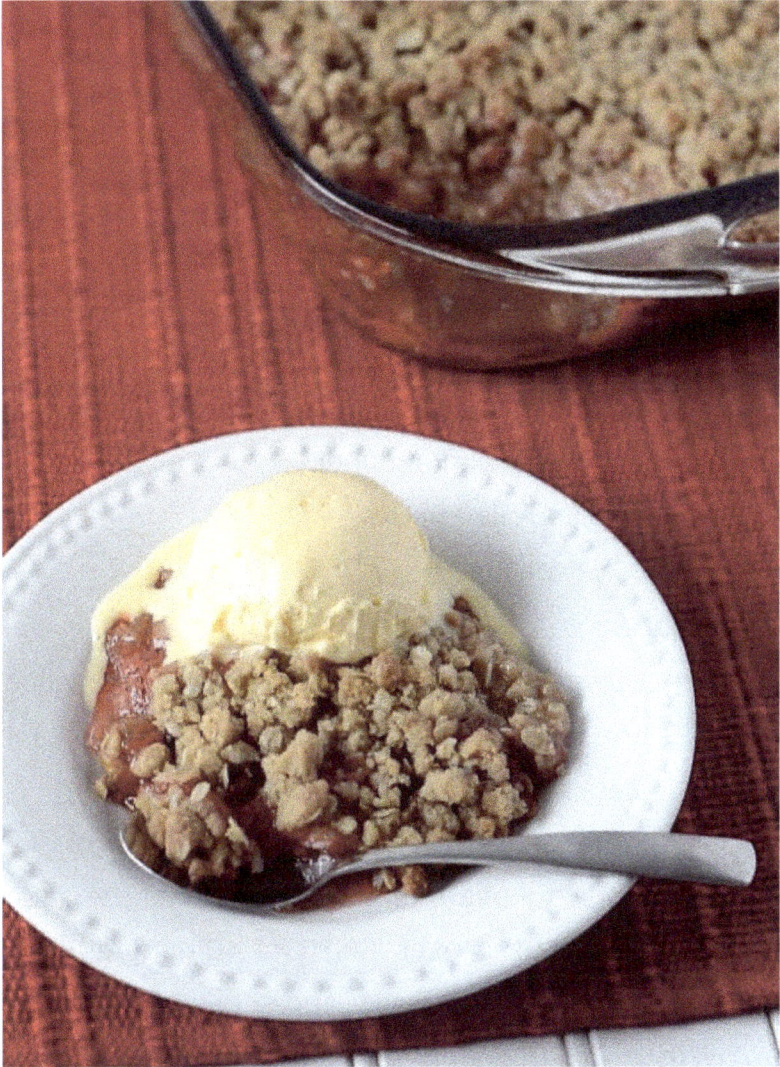

Cranberries and Pears Pie

Preparation Time: 10 minutes

Cooking Time: 40 minutes

Servings: 4

Ingredients:

- 2 cup cranberries
- 3 cups pears, cubed
- A drizzle of olive oil
- 1 cup stevia
- 1/3 cup almond flour
- 1 cup rolled oats
- ¼ avocado oil

Directions:

1. In a bowl, mix the cranberries with the pears and the other ingredients except the olive oil and the oats, and stir well.
2. Grease a cake pan with the a drizzle of olive oil, pour the pears mix inside, sprinkle the oats all over and bake at 350°F for 40 minutes.
3. Cool the mix down, and serve.

Nutrition:

Calories 172

Fat 3.4g

Carbs 11.5g

Protein 4.5g

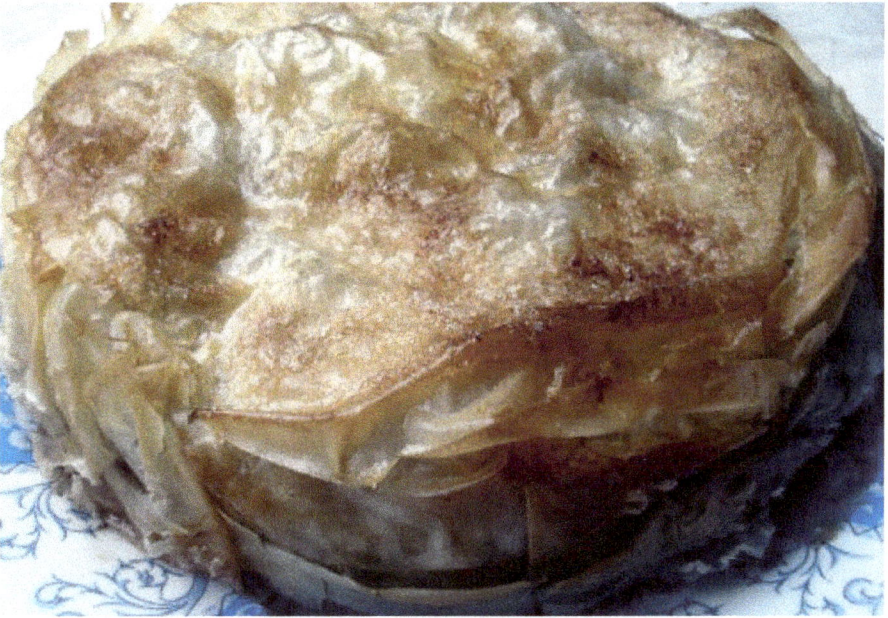

Lemon Cream

Preparation Time: 1 hour

Cooking Time: 10 minutes

Servings: 6

Ingredients:

- 2 eggs, whisked
- 1 and ¼ cup stevia
- 10 tbsp. avocado oil
- 1 cup heavy cream
- Juice of 2 lemons
- Zest of 2 lemons, grated

Directions:

In a pan, combine the cream with the lemon juice and the other ingredients, whisk well, cook for 10 minutes, divide into cups and keep in the fridge for 1 hour before serving.

Nutrition:

Calories 200

Fat 8.5g

Carbs 8.6g

Protein 4.5g

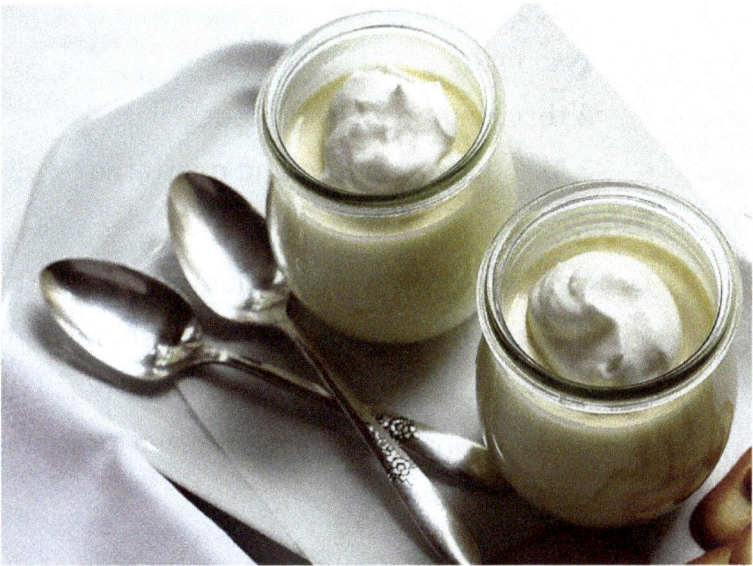

Peach Sorbet

Preparation Time: 2 hours

Cooking Time: 10 minutes

Servings: 4

Ingredients:

- 2 cups apple juice
- 1 cup stevia
- 2 tbsp. lemon zest, grated
- 2 lb. peaches, pitted and quartered

Directions:

1. Heat up a pan over medium heat, add the apple juice and the rest of the ingredients, simmer for 10 minutes, transfer to a blender, pulse, divide into cups and keep in the freezer for 2 hours before serving.

Nutrition:

Calories 182

Fat 5.4g

Carbs 12g

Protein 5.4g

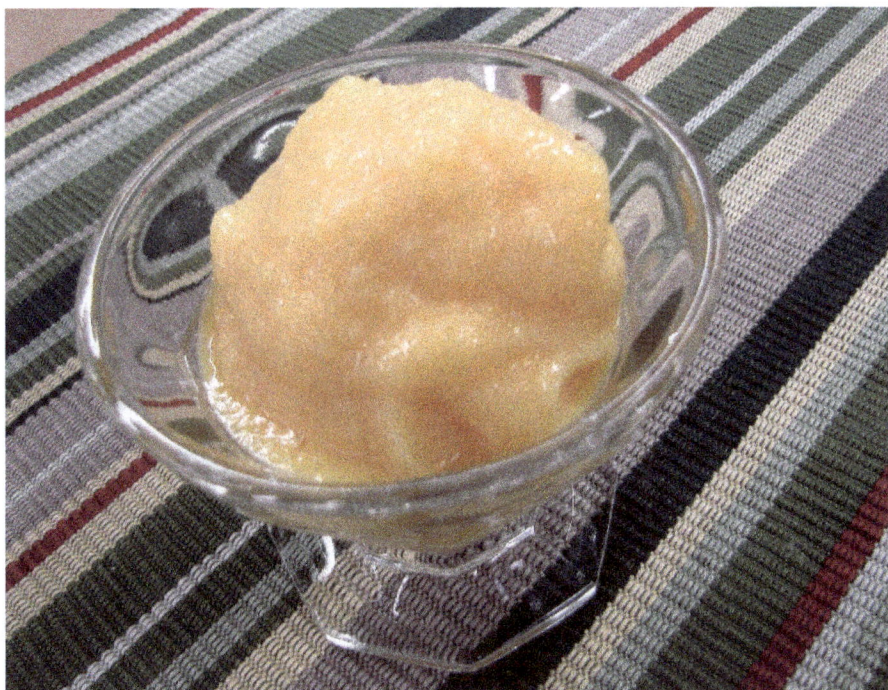

Almond Rice Dessert

Preparation Time: 10 minutes

Cooking Time: 20 minutes

Servings: 4

Ingredients:

- 1 cup white rice
- 2 cups almond milk
- 1 cup almonds, chopped
- ½ cup stevia
- 1 tbsp. cinnamon powder
- ½ cup pomegranate seeds

Directions:

1. In a pot, mix the rice with the milk and stevia, bring to a simmer and cook for 20 minutes, stirring often.
2. Add the rest of the ingredients, stir, divide into bowls and serve.

Nutrition:

Calories 234

Fat 9.5g

Carbs 12.4g

Protein 6.5g

Blueberries Stew

Preparation Time: 10 minutes

Cooking Time: 10 minutes

Servings: 4

Ingredients:

- 2 cups blueberries
- 3 tbsp. stevia
- 1 and ½ cups pure apple juice
- 1 tsp. vanilla extract

Directions:

1. In a pan, combine the blueberries with stevia and the other ingredients, bring to a simmer and cook over medium-low heat for 10 minutes.
2. Divide into cups and serve cold.

Nutrition:

Calories 192

Fat 5.4g

Carbs 9.4g

Protein 4.5g

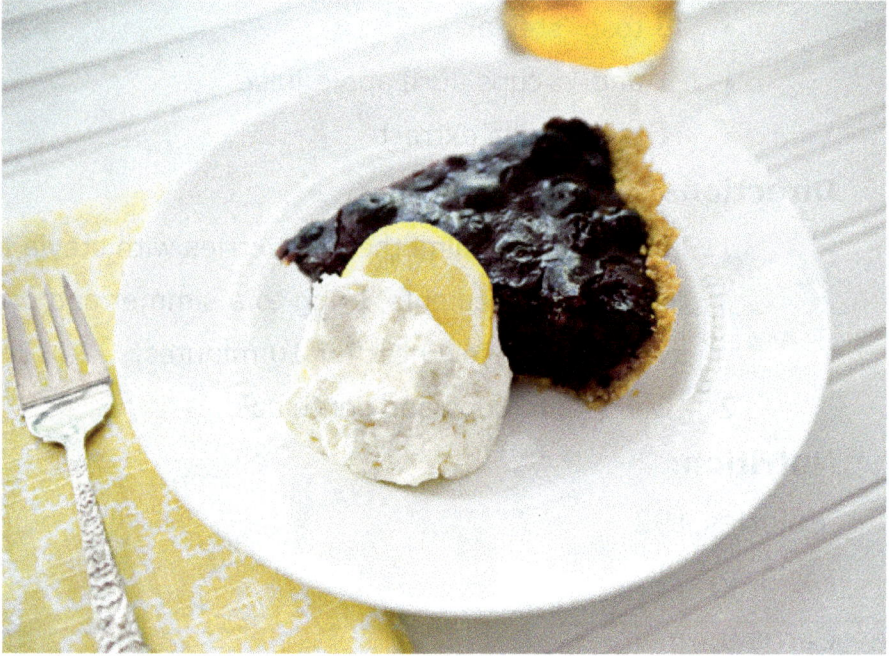

Mandarin Cream

Preparation Time: 20 minutes

Cooking Time: 0 minutes

Servings: 8

Ingredients:

- 2 mandarins, peeled and cut into segments
- Juice of 2 mandarins
- 2 tbsp. stevia
- 4 eggs, whisked
- ¾ cup stevia
- ¾ cup almonds, ground

Directions:

1. In a blender, combine the mandarins with the mandarin's juice and the other ingredients, whisk well, divide into cups and keep in the fridge for 20 minutes before serving.

Nutrition:

Calories 106

Fat 3.4g

Carbs 2.4g

Protein 4g

Creamy Mint Strawberry Mix

Preparation Time: 10 minutes

Cooking Time: 30 minutes

Servings: 6

Ingredients:

- Cooking spray
- ¼ cup stevia
- 1 and ½ cup almond flour
- 1 tsp. baking powder
- 1 cup almond milk
- 1 egg, whisked
- 2 cups strawberries, sliced
- 1 tbsp. mint, chopped
- 1 tsp. lime zest, grated
- ½ cup whipping cream

Directions:

1. In a bowl, combine the almond with the strawberries, mint and the other ingredients except the cooking spray and whisk well.
2. Grease 6 ramekins with the cooking spray, pour the strawberry mix inside, introduce in the oven and bake at 350°F for 30 minutes.
3. Cool down and serve.

Nutrition:

Calories 200

Fat 6.3g

Carbs 6.5g

Protein 8g

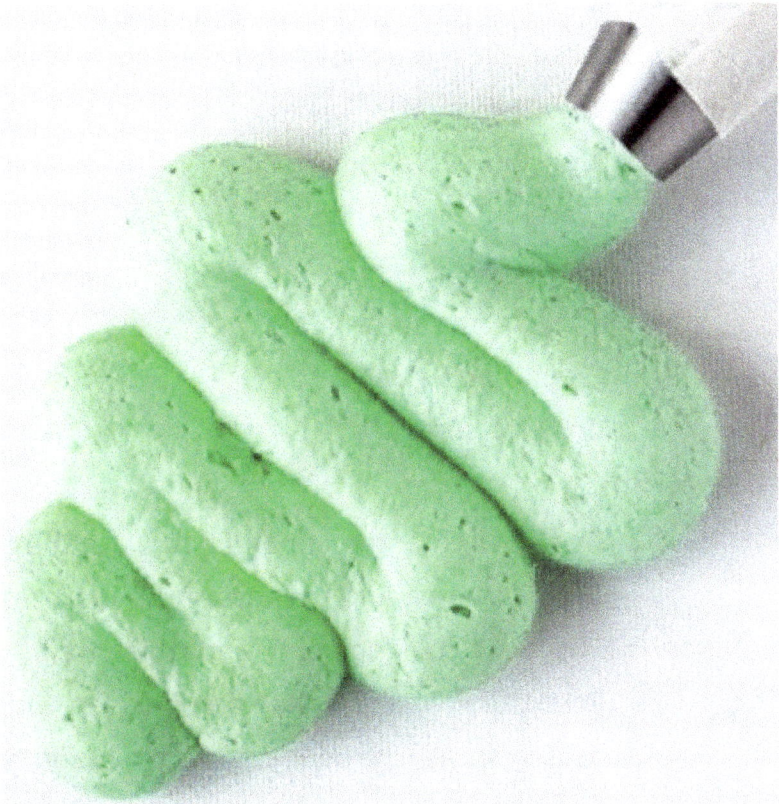

Vanilla Cake

Preparation Time: 10 minutes

Cooking Time: 25 minutes

Servings: 10

Ingredients:

- 3 cups almond flour
- 3 tsp. baking powder
- 1 cup olive oil
- 1 and ½ cup almond milk
- 1 and 2/3 cup stevia
- 2 cups water
- 1 tbsp. lime juice
- 2 tsp. vanilla extract
- Cooking spray

Directions:

1. In a bowl, mix the almond flour with the baking powder, the oil and the rest of the ingredients except the cooking spray and whisk well.
2. Pour the mix into a cake pan greased with the cooking spray, introduce in the oven and bake at 370°F for 25 minutes.
3. Leave the cake to cool down, cut and serve!

Nutrition:

Calories 200

Fat 7.6g

Carbs 5.5g

Protein 4.5g

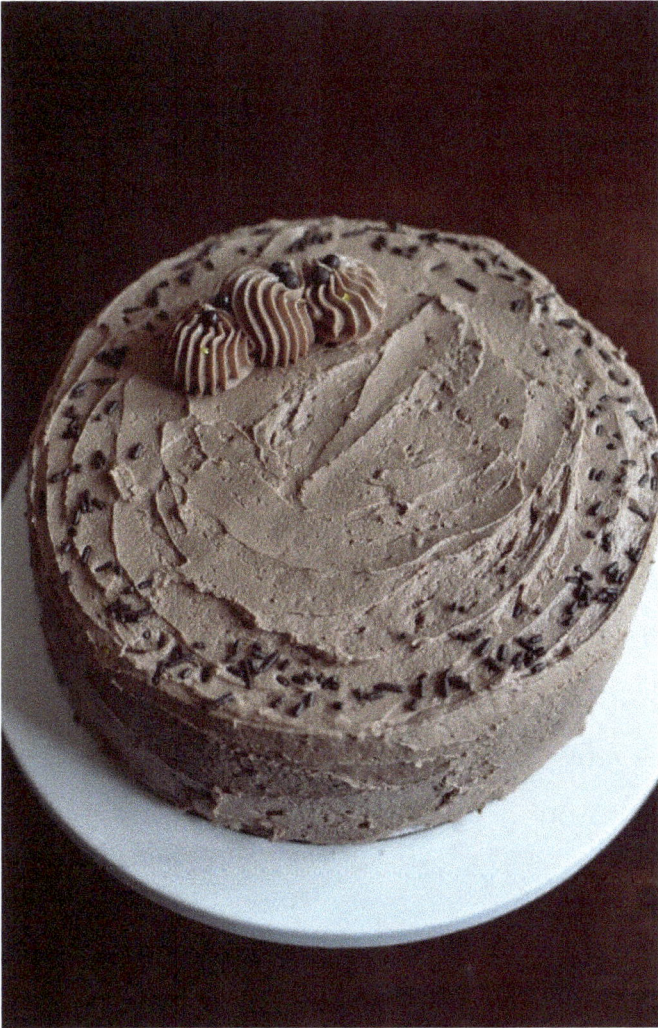

Pumpkin Cream

Preparation Time: 5 minutes

Cooking Time: 5 minutes

Servings: 2

Ingredients:

- 2 cups canned pumpkin flesh
- 2 tbsp. stevia
- 1 tsp. vanilla extract
- 2 tbsp. water
- A pinch of pumpkin spice

Directions:

1. In a pan, combine the pumpkin flesh with the other ingredients, simmer for 5 minutes, divide into cups and serve cold.

Nutrition:

Calories 192

Fat 3.4g

Carbs 7.6g

Protein 3.5g

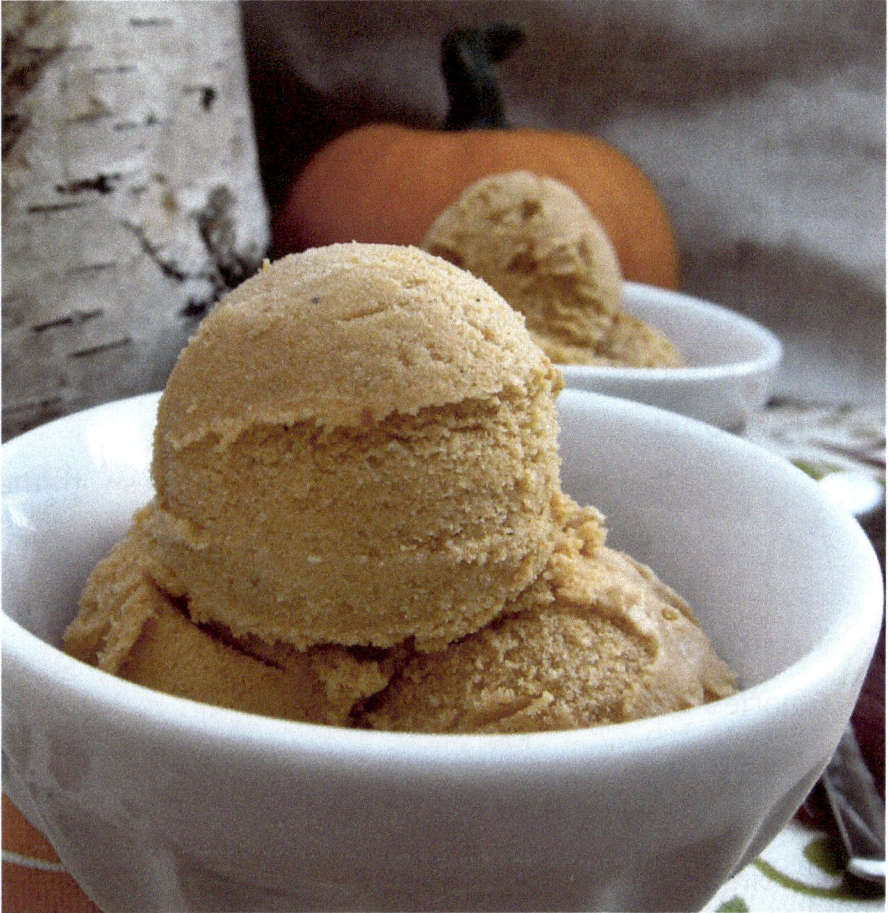

Chia and Berries Smoothie Bowl

Preparation Time: 5 minutes

Cooking Time: 0 minutes

Servings: 2

Ingredients:

- 1 and ½ cup almond milk
- 1 cup blackberries
- ¼ cup strawberries, chopped
- 1 and ½ tbsp. chia seeds
- 1 tsp. cinnamon powder

Directions:

1. In a blender, combine the blackberries with the strawberries and the rest of the ingredients, pulse well, divide into small bowls and serve cold.

Nutrition:

Calories 182

Fat 3.4g

Carbs 8.4g

Protein 3g

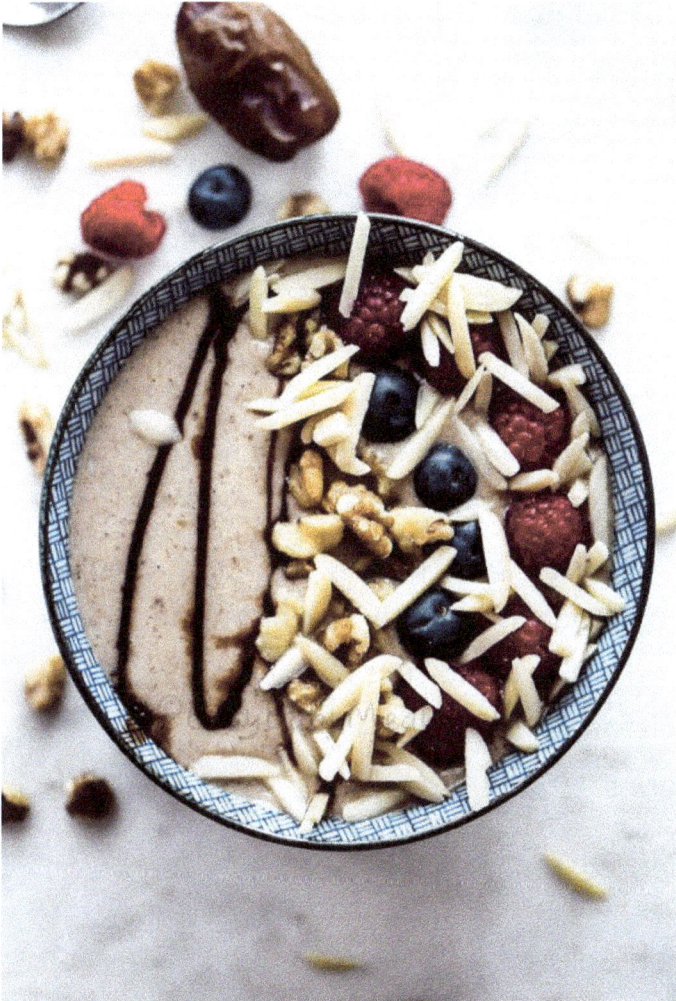

Minty Coconut Cream

Preparation Time: 4 minutes

Cooking Time: 0 minutes

Servings: 2

Ingredients:

- 1 banana, peeled
- 2 cups coconut flesh, shredded
- 3 tbsp. mint, chopped
- 1 and ½ cups coconut water
- 2 tbsp. stevia
- ½ avocado, pitted and peeled

Directions:

1. In a blender, combine the coconut with the banana and the rest of the ingredients, pulse well, divide into cups and serve cold.

Nutrition:

Calories 193

Fat 5.4g

Carbs 7.6g

Protein 3g

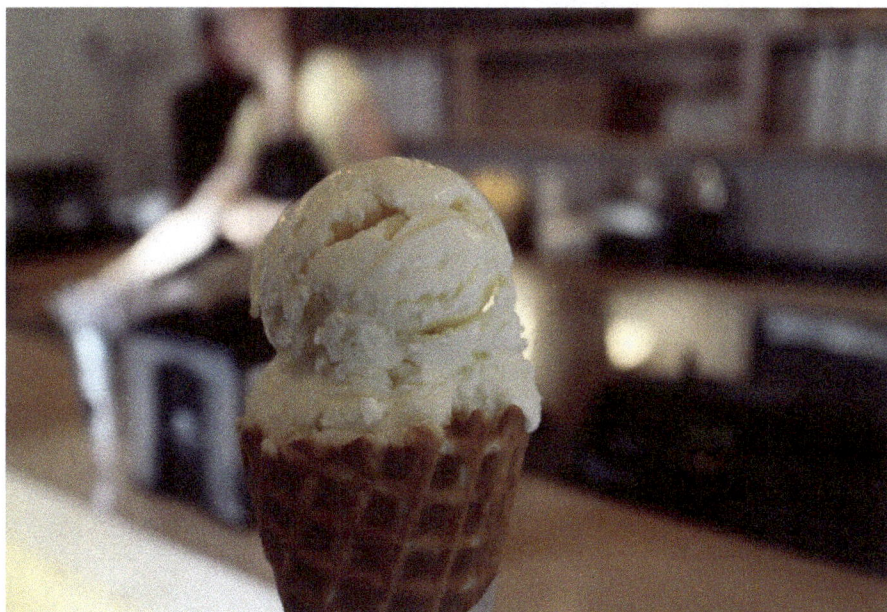

Watermelon Cream

Preparation Time: 15 minutes

Cooking Time: 0 minutes

Servings: 2

Ingredients:

- 1-lb. watermelon, peeled and chopped
- 1 tsp. vanilla extract
- 1 cup heavy cream
- 1 tsp. lime juice
- 2 tbsp. stevia

Directions:

1. In a blender, combine the watermelon with the cream and the rest of the ingredients, pulse well, divide into cups and keep in the fridge for 15 minutes before serving.

Nutrition:

Calories 122

Fat 5.7

Carbs 5.3

Protein 0.4

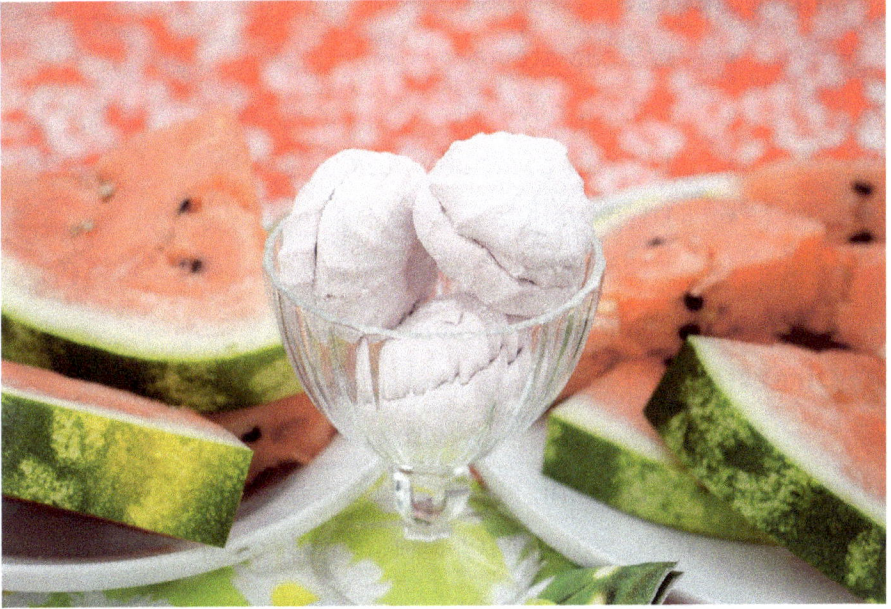

Grapes Stew

Preparation Time: 10 minutes

Cooking Time: 10 minutes

Servings: 4

Ingredients:

- 2/3 cup stevia
- 1 tbsp. olive oil
- 1/3 cup coconut water
- 1 tsp. vanilla extract
- 1 tsp. lemon zest, grated
- 2 cup red grapes, halved

Directions:

1. Heat up a pan with the water over medium heat, add the oil, stevia and the rest of the ingredients, toss, simmer for 10 minutes, divide into cups and serve.

Nutrition:

Calories 122

Fat 3.7

Carbs 2.3

Protein 0.4

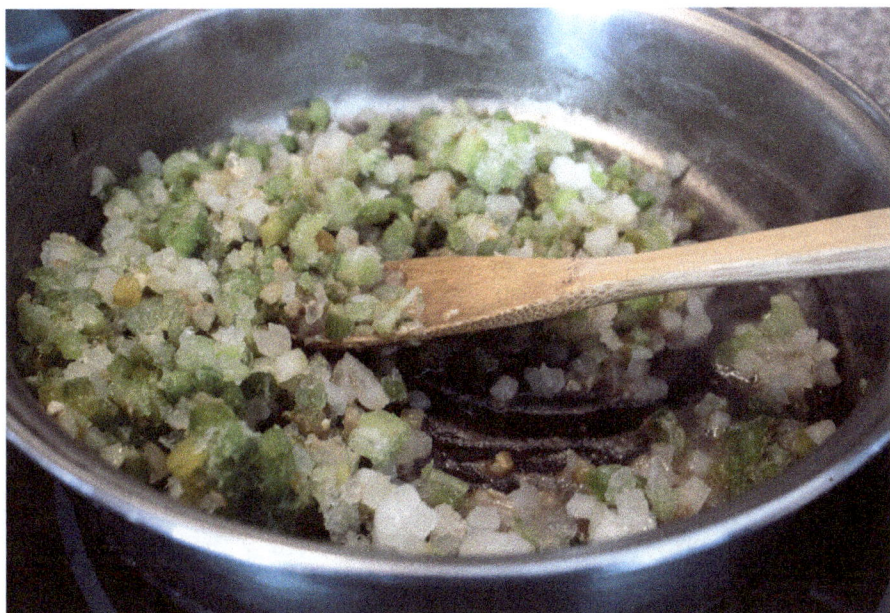

Cocoa Sweet Cherry Cream

Preparation Time: 2 hours

Cooking Time: 0 minutes

Servings: 4

Ingredients:

- ½ cup cocoa powder
- ¾ cup red cherry jam
- ¼ cup stevia
- 2 cups water
- 1-lb. cherries, pitted and halved

Directions:

1. In a blender, mix the cherries with the water and the rest of the ingredients, pulse well, divide into cups and keep in the fridge for 2 hours before serving.

Nutrition:

Calories 162

Fat 3.4g

Carbs 5g

Protein 1g

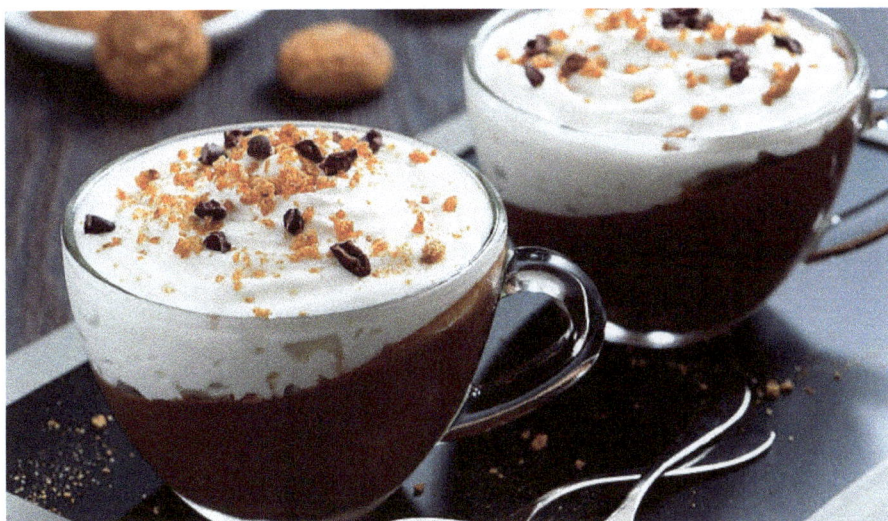

Apple Couscous Pudding

Preparation Time: 10 minutes

Cooking Time: 25 minutes

Servings: 4

Ingredients:

- ½ cup couscous
- 1 and ½ cups milk
- ¼ cup apple, cored and chopped
- 3 tbsp. stevia
- ½ tsp. rose water
- 1 tbsp. orange zest, grated

Directions:

1. Heat up a pan with the milk over medium heat, add the couscous and the rest of the ingredients, whisk, simmer for 25 minutes, divide into bowls and serve.

Nutrition:

Calories 150

Fat 4.5g

Carbs 7.5g

Protein 4g

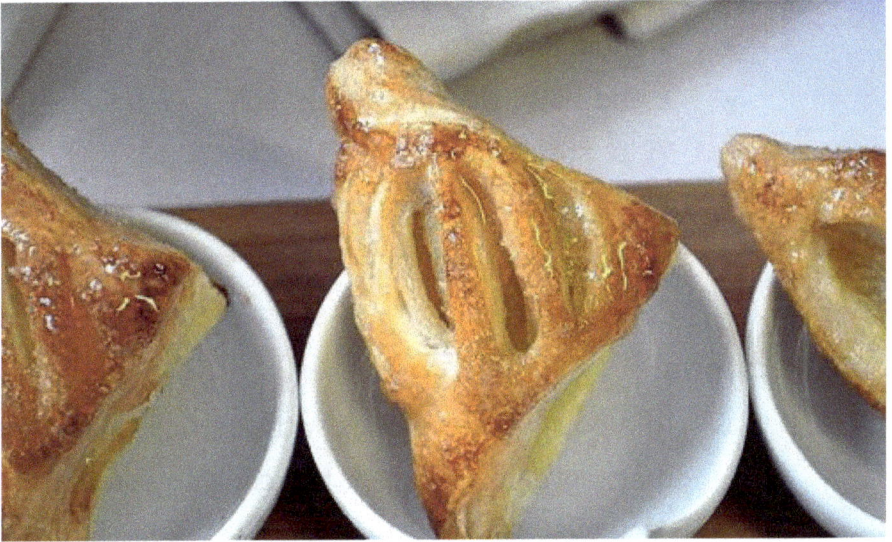

Ricotta Ramekins

Preparation Time: 10 minutes

Cooking Time: 1 hour

Servings: 4

Ingredients:

- 6 eggs, whisked
- 1 and ½ lb. ricotta cheese, soft
- ½ lb. stevia
- 1 tsp. vanilla extract
- ½ tsp. baking powder
- Cooking spray

Directions:

1. In a bowl, mix the eggs with the ricotta and the other ingredients except the cooking spray and whisk well.
2. Grease 4 ramekins with the cooking spray, pour the ricotta cream in each and bake at 360°F for 1 hour.
3. Serve cold.

Nutrition:

Calories 180

Fat 5.3g

Carbs 11.5g

Protein 4g

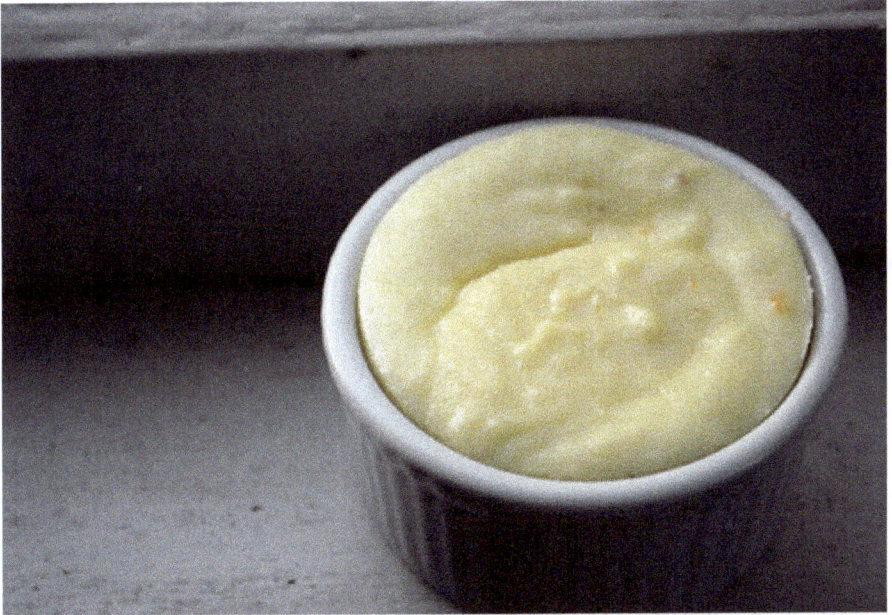

Papaya Cream

Preparation Time: 10 minutes

Cooking Time: 0 minutes

Servings: 2

Ingredients:

- 1 cup papaya, peeled and chopped
- 1 cup heavy cream
- 1 tbsp. stevia
- ½ tsp. vanilla extract

Directions:

1. In a blender, combine the cream with the papaya and the other ingredients, pulse well, divide into cups and serve cold.

Nutrition:

Calories 182

Fiber 2.3g

Carbs 3.5g

Protein 2g

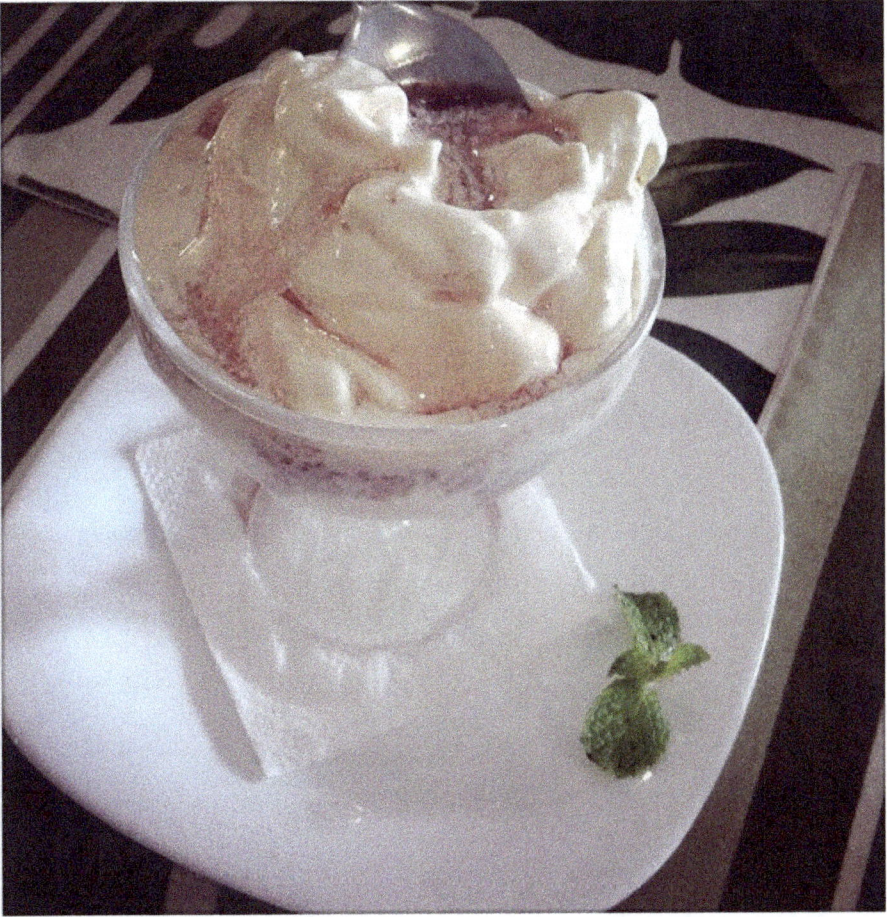

Almonds and Oats Pudding

Preparation Time: 10 minutes

Cooking Time: 15 minutes

Servings: 4

Ingredients:

- 1 tbsp. lemon juice
- Zest of 1 lime
- 1 and ½ cups almond milk
- 1 tsp. almond extract
- ½ cup oats
- 2 tbsp. stevia
- ½ cup silver almonds, chopped

Directions:

1. In a pan, combine the almond milk with the lime zest and the other ingredients, whisk, bring to a

simmer and cook over medium heat for 15 minutes.

2. Divide the mix into bowls and serve cold.

Nutrition:

Calories 174

Fat 12.1g

Carbs 3.9g

Protein 4.8g

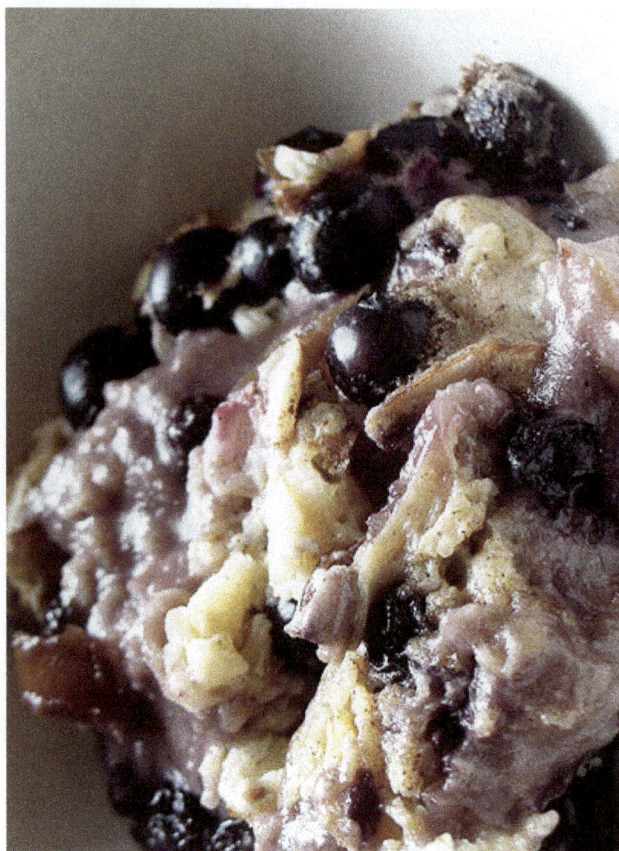

Strawberry Sorbet

Preparation Time: 15 minutes

Cooking Time: 10 minutes

Servings: 6

Ingredients:

- 1 cup strawberries, chopped
- 1 tbsp. of liquid honey
- 2 tbsp. water
- 1 tbsp. lemon juice

Directions:

1. Preheat the water and liquid honey until you get homogenous liquid.
2. Blend the strawberries until smooth and combine them with honey liquid and lemon juice.

3. Transfer the strawberry mixture in the ice cream maker and churn it for 20 minutes or until the sorbet is thick.

4. Scoop the cooked sorbet in the ice cream cups.

Nutrition:

Calories 30,

Fat 0.4 g,

Carbs 14.9 g,

Protein 0.9 g

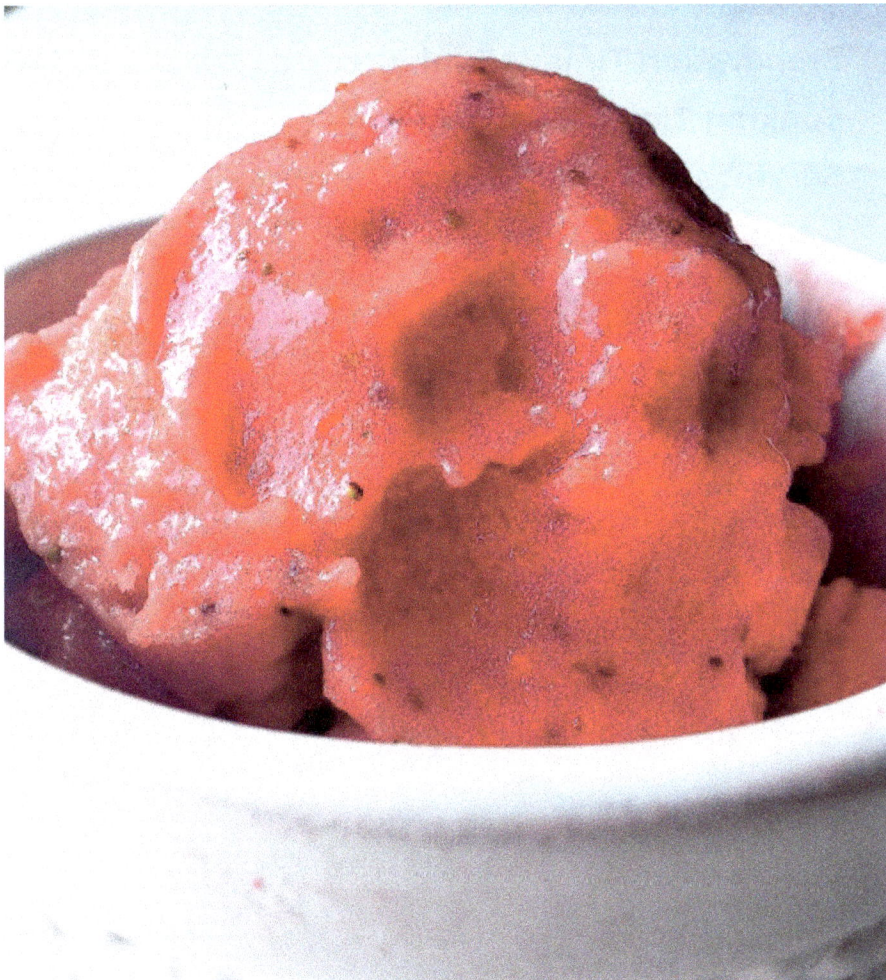

Vanilla Apple Pie

Preparation Time: 15 minutes
Cooking Time: 50 minutes
Servings: 8

Ingredients:

- 3 apples, sliced
- ½ tsp. ground cinnamon
- 1 tsp. vanilla extract
- 1 tbsp. Erythritol
- 7 oz yeast roll dough
- 1 egg, beaten

Directions:

1. Roll up the dough and cut it on 2 parts.
2. Line the springform pan with baking paper.
3. Place the first dough part in the springform pan.

4. Then arrange the apples over the dough and sprinkle it with Erythritol, vanilla extract, and ground cinnamon.

5. Then cover the apples with remaining dough and secure the edges of the pie with the help of the fork.

6. Make the small cuts in the surface of the pie.

7. Brush the pie with beaten egg and bake it for 50 minutes at 375°F.

8. Cool the cooked pie well and then remove from the springform pan.

9. Cut it on the servings.

Nutrition:

Calories 140,

Fat 3.4 g,

Carbs 23.9 g,

Protein 2.9 g

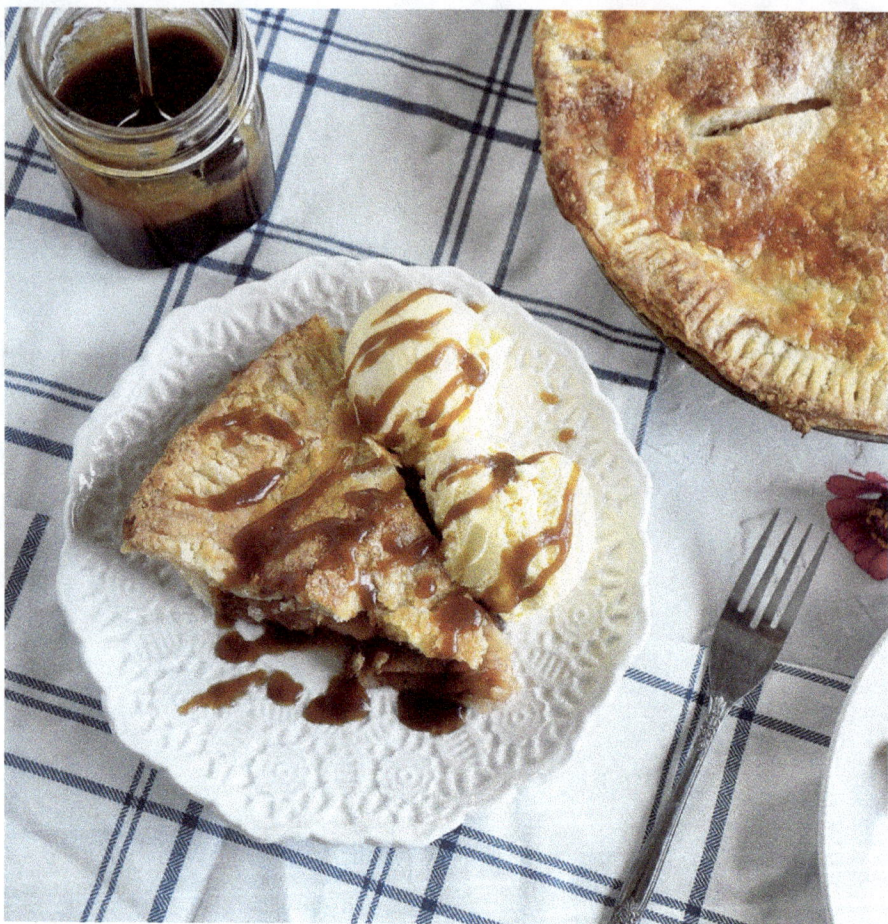

Cinnamon Pears

Preparation Time: 2 hours

Cooking Time: 0 minutes

Servings: 6

Ingredients:

- 2 pears
- 1 tsp. ground cinnamon
- 1 tbsp. Erythritol
- 1 tsp. liquid stevia
- 4 tsp. butter

Directions:

1. Cut the pears on the halves.
2. Then scoop the seeds from the pears with the help of the scooper.
3. In the shallow bowl mix up together Erythritol and ground cinnamon.

4. Sprinkle every pear half with cinnamon mixture and drizzle with liquid stevia.
5. Then add butter and wrap in the foil.
6. Bake the pears for 25 minutes at 365°F.
7. Then remove the pears from the foil and transfer in the serving plates.

Nutrition:

Calories 96,

Fat 4.4 g,

Carbs 3.9 g,

Protein 0.9 g

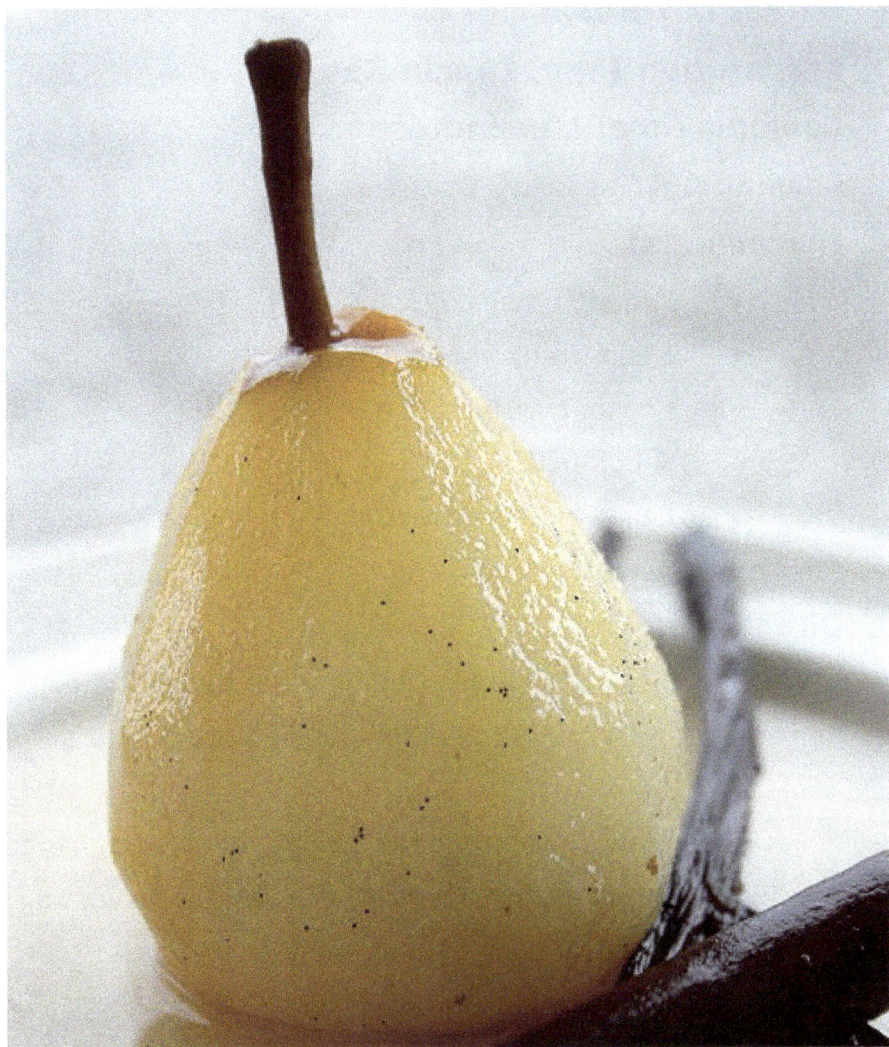

Ginger Ice Cream

Preparation Time: 15 minutes

Cooking Time: 10 minutes

Servings: 6

Ingredients:

- 1 mango, peeled
- 1 cup Greek yogurt
- 1 tbsp. Erythritol
- ¼ cup milk
- 1 tsp. vanilla extract
- ¼ tsp. ground ginger

Directions:

1. Blend the mango until you get puree and combine it with Erythritol, milk, vanilla extract, and ground ginger.
2. Then mix up together Greek yogurt and mango puree mixture. Transfer it in the plastic vessel.
3. Freeze the ice cream for 35 minutes.

Nutrition:

Calories 90,

Fat 1.4 g,

Carbs 21.9 g,

Protein 4.9 g

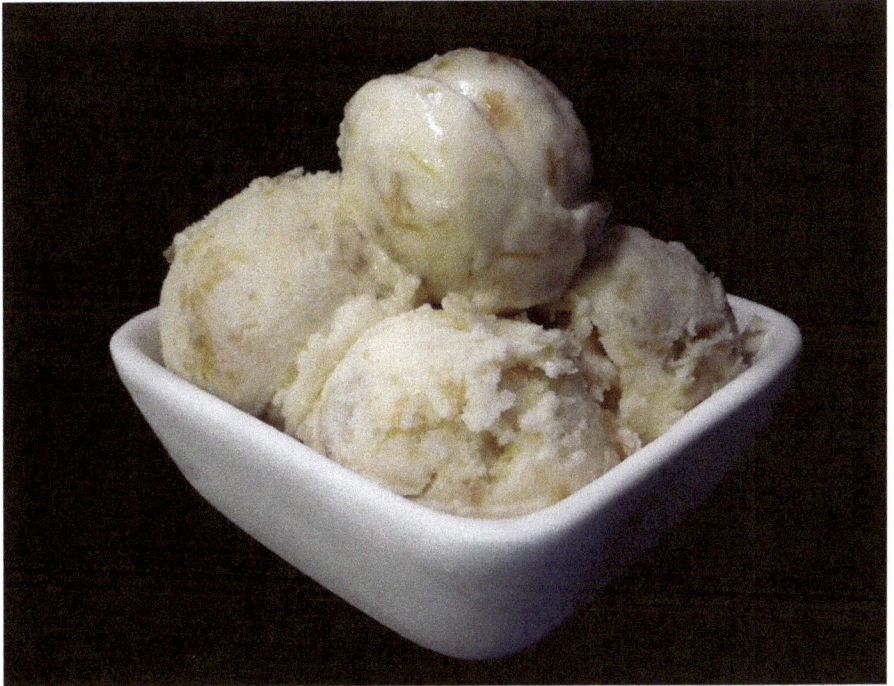

Cherry Compote

Preparation Time: 2 hours

Cooking Time: 0 minutes

Servings: 6

Ingredients:

- 2 peaches, pitted, halved
- 1 cup cherries, pitted
- ½ cup grape juice
- ½ cup strawberries
- 1 tbsp. liquid honey
- 1 tsp. vanilla extract
- 1 tsp. ground cinnamon

Directions:

1. Pour grape juice in the saucepan.
2. Add vanilla extract and ground cinnamon. Bring the liquid to boil.

3. After this, put peaches, cherries, and strawberries in the hot grape juice and bring to boil.
4. Remove the mixture from heat, add liquid honey, and close the lid.
5. Let the compote rest for 20 minutes.
6. Carefully mix up the compote and transfer in the serving plate.

Nutrition:

Calories 80,

Fat 0.4 g,

Carbs 19.9 g,

Protein 0.9 g

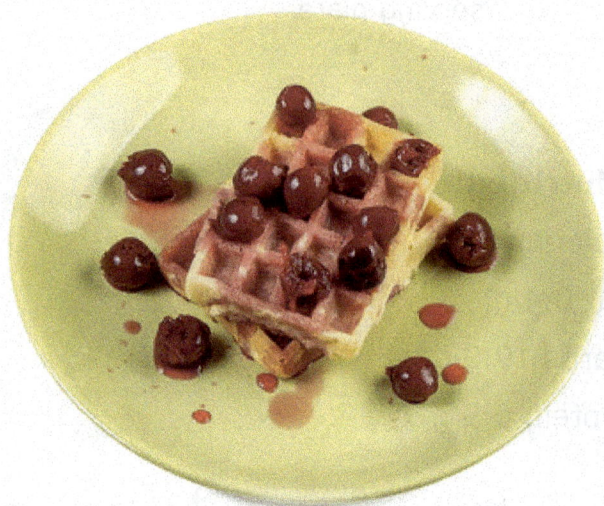

Creamy Strawberries

Preparation Time: 15 minutes

Cooking Time: 10 minutes

Servings: 6

Ingredients:

- 6 tbsp. almond butter
- 1 tbsp. Erythritol
- 1 cup milk
- 1 tsp. vanilla extract
- 1 cup strawberries, sliced

Directions:

1. Pour milk in the saucepan.
2. Add Erythritol, vanilla extract, and almond butter.
3. With the help of the hand mixer mix up the liquid until smooth and bring it to boil.

4. Then remove the mixture from the heat and let it cool.
5. The cooled mixture will be thick.
6. Put the strawberries in the serving glasses and top with the thick almond butter dip.

Nutrition:

Calories 192,

Fat 14.4 g,

Carbs 10.9 g,

Protein 1.9 g

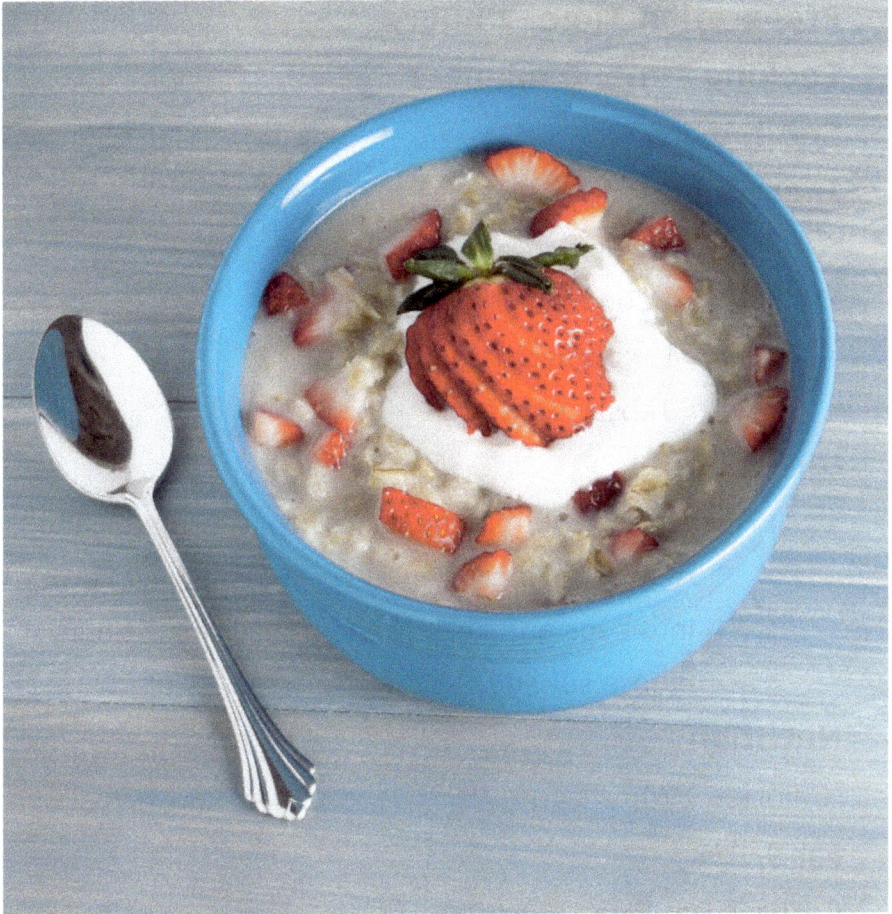

Chocolate Cups

Preparation Time: 2 hours

Cooking Time: 0 minutes

Servings: 6

Ingredients:

- ½ cup avocado oil
- 1 cup, chocolate, melted
- 1 tsp. matcha powder
- 3 tbsp. stevia

Directions:

1. In a bowl, mix the chocolate with the oil and the rest of the ingredients, whisk really well, divide into cups and keep in the freezer for 2 hours before serving.

Nutrition:

Calories 174

Fat 9.1g

Carbs 3.9g

Protein 2.8g

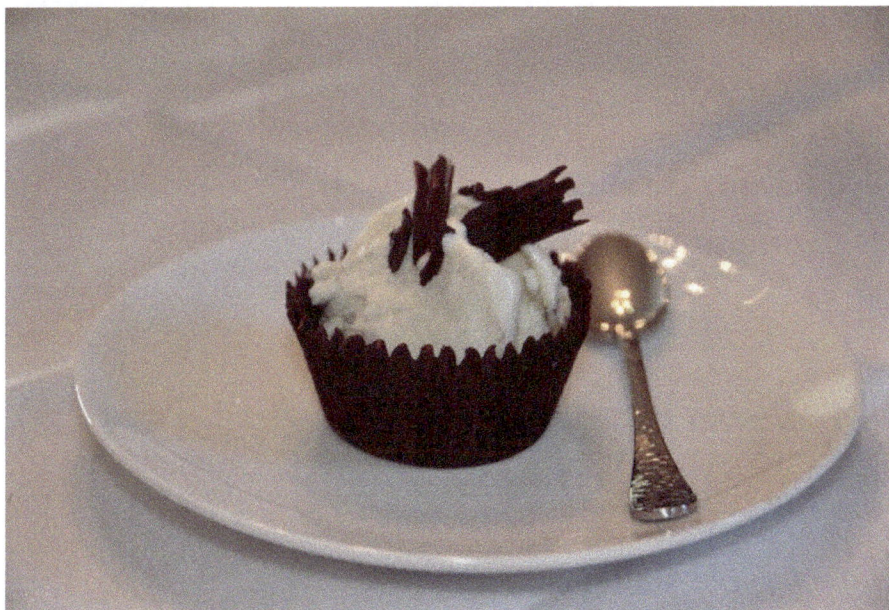

Honey Walnut Bars

Preparation Time: 20 minutes

Cooking Time: 30 minutes

Servings: 8

Ingredients:

- 5 oz puff pastry
- ½ cup of water
- 3 tbsp. of liquid honey
- 1 tsp. Erythritol
- 1/3 cup butter, softened
- ½ cup walnuts, chopped
- 1 tsp. olive oil

Directions:

1. Roll up the puff pastry and cut it on 6 sheets.
2. Then brush the tray with olive oil and arrange the first puff pastry sheet inside.

3. Grease it with butter gently and sprinkle with walnuts.
4. Repeat the same steps with 4 puff pastry sheets.
5. Then sprinkle the last layer with walnuts and Erythritol and cove with the sixth puff pastry sheet.
6. Cut the baklava on the servings.
7. Bake the baklava for 30 minutes.
8. Meanwhile, bring to boil liquid honey and water.
9. When the baklava is cooked, remove it from the oven.
10. Pour hot honey liquid over baklava and let it cool till the room temperature.

Nutrition:

Calories 243,

Fat 4.4 g,

Carbs 15.9 g,

Protein 1.9 g

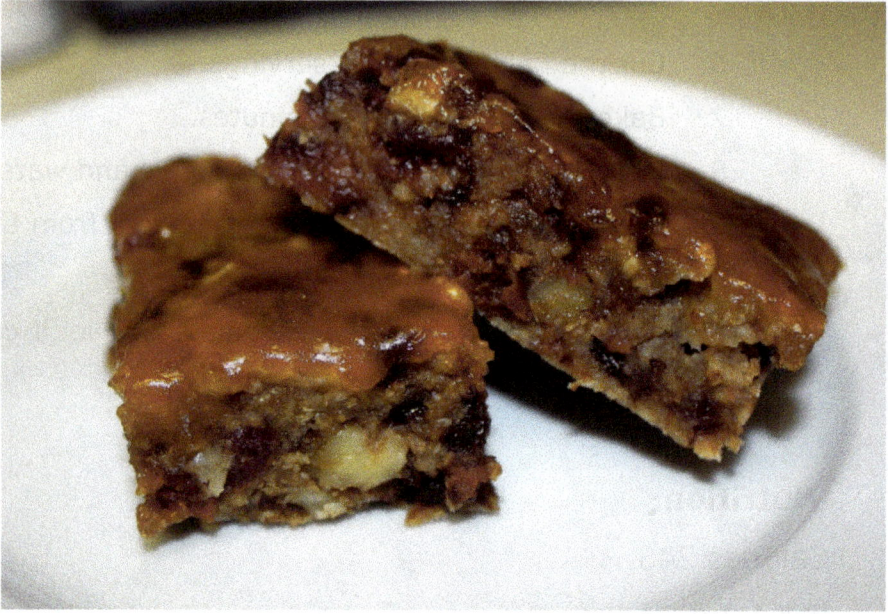

Yogurt Parfait

Preparation Time: 5 minutes

Cooking Time: 0 minutes

Servings: 1

Ingredients:

- 1 oz blueberries
- 2 tbsp. Plain yogurt
- ½ tsp. vanilla extract

Directions:

1. Mix up together Plain yogurt and vanilla extract.
2. Then put ½ oz of blueberries in the glass.
3. Cover the berries with ½ part of Plain Yogurt.
4. Then add the layer of berries.
5. Top parfait with remaining Plain yogurt.

Nutrition:

Calories 44,

Fat 0.4 g,

Carbs 6.9 g,

Protein 1.9 g

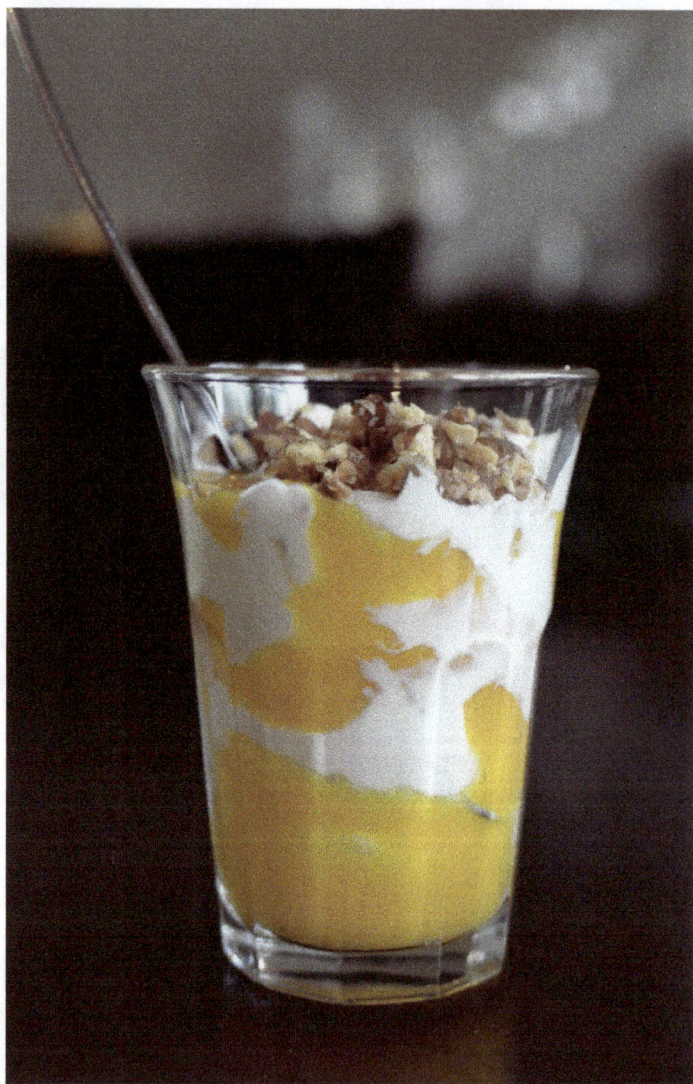

Raspberry Tart

Preparation Time: 15 minutes

Cooking Time: 10 minutes

Servings: 6

Ingredients:

- 3 tbsp. butter, softened
- 1 cup wheat flour, whole wheat
- 1 tsp. baking powder
- 1 egg, beaten
- 4 tbsp. pistachio paste
- 2 tbsp. raspberry jam

Directions:

1. Knead the dough: combine together softened butter, flour, baking powder, and egg. You should get the non-sticky and very soft dough.

2. Put the dough in the springform pan and flatten it with the help of the fingertips until you get pie crust.
3. Bake it for 10 minutes at 365°F.
4. After this, spread the pie crust with raspberry jam and then with pistachio paste.
5. Bake the tart at 365°F for another 10 minutes.
6. Cool the cooked tart and cut on the servings.

Nutrition:

Calories 311,

Fat 11.4 g,

Carbs 14.9 g,

Protein 1.9 g

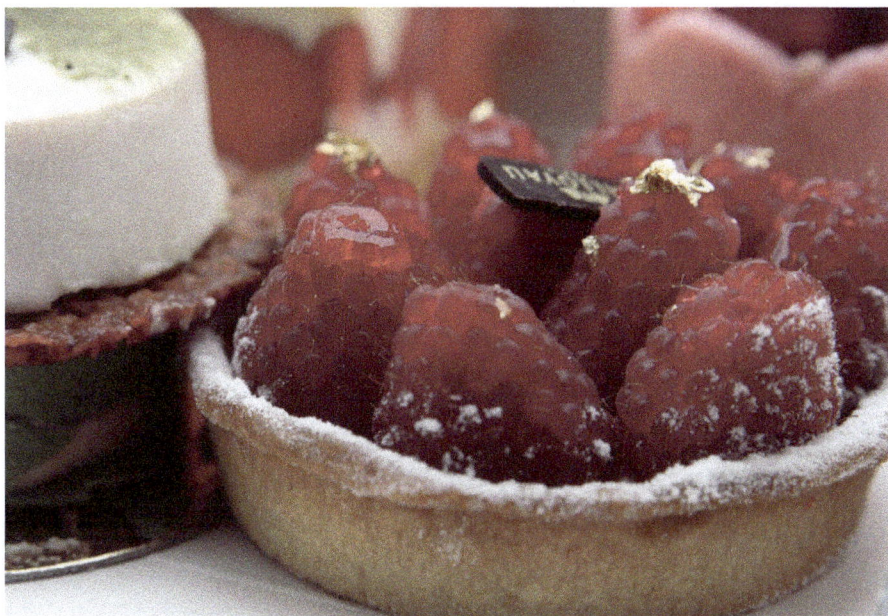

Quinoa Energy Bars

Preparation Time: 20 minutes

Cooking Time: 15 minutes

Servings: 8

Ingredients:

- ½ cup puffed quinoa
- ¼ cup oats
- 2 oz dark chocolate
- 2 tbsp. almond butter
- ¾ cup maple syrup
- 1 tbsp. butter
- 1 tbsp. coconut flakes

Directions:

1. Place dark chocolate, butter, maple syrup, and almond butter in the saucepan.
2. Melt the mixture and add oats, puffed quinoa, and coconut flakes.

3. Mix up well and remove it from the heat.

4. After this, line the baking tray with baking paper and transfer the quinoa mixture in it.

5. Flatten it well with the help of the spatula and cut on the bars (8 pieces).

6. Bake the quinoa bars for 10 minutes at 365°F.

7. After this, remove the tray with quinoa bars from the oven and cool well.

Nutrition:

Calories 240,

Fat 6.4 g,

Carbs 29.9 g,

Protein 1.9 g

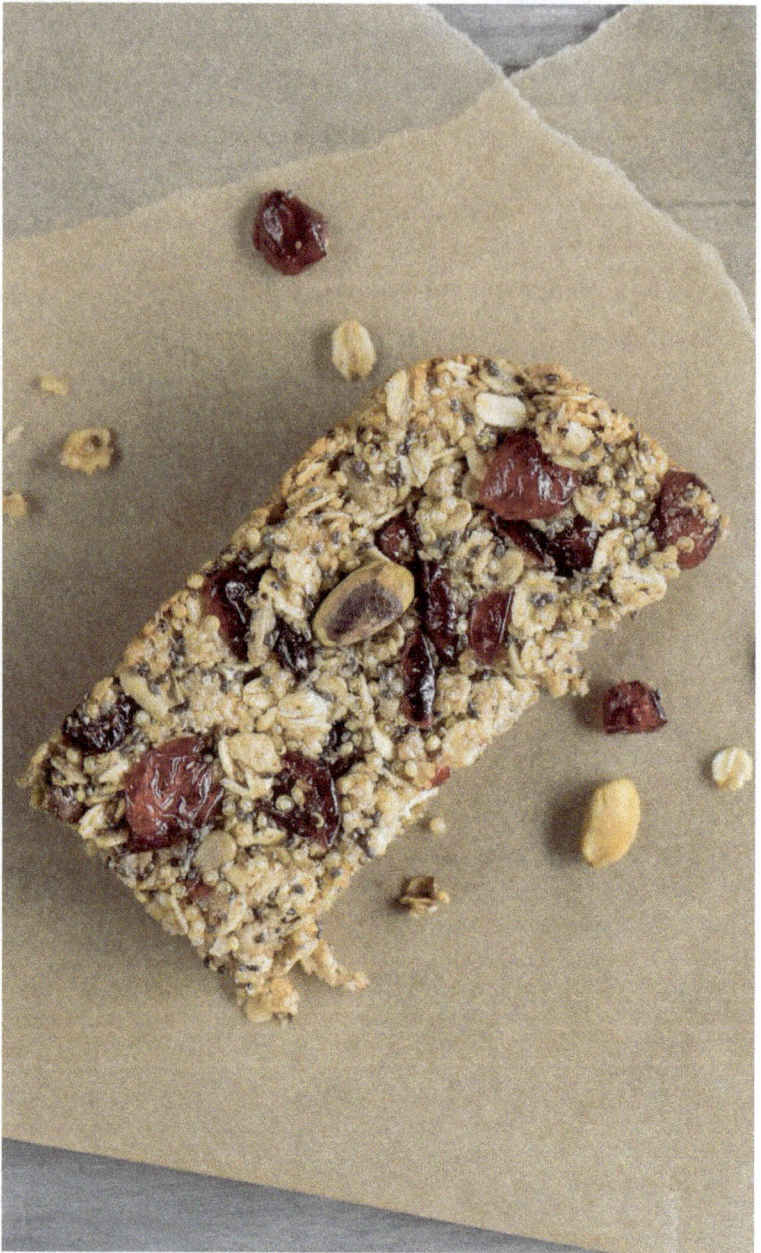

www.ingramcontent.com/pod-product-compliance
Lightning Source LLC
Chambersburg PA
CBHW050751030426
42336CB00012B/1770